FUNDAMENTALS OF VISCERAL INNERVATION

FUNDAMENTALS OF VISCERAL INNERVATION

By

BUDH DEV BHAGAT

Professor of Physiology and Pharmacology
Saint Louis University
School of Medicine
St. Louis, Missouri

PAUL A. YOUNG

Professor of Anatomy
Saint Louis University
School of Medicine
St. Louis, Missouri

DONALD E. BIGGERSTAFF

Chief, Medical Illustration
Southern Illinois University
School of Medicine
Springfield, Illinois

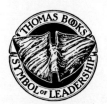

CHARLES C THOMAS • PUBLISHER
Springfield • Illinois • U.S.A.

Published and Distributed Throughout the World by

CHARLES C THOMAS • PUBLISHER
Bannerstone House
301-327 East Lawrence Avenue, Springfield, Illinois, U.S.A.

© *1977, by* CHARLES C THOMAS • PUBLISHER

ISBN 0-398-03388-9 (cloth)
0-398-03390-0 (paper)

Library of Congress Catalog Card Number: 74-30208

Printed in the United States of America

BB-14

Library of Congress Cataloging in Publication Data

Bhagat, Budh Dev.
    Fundamentals of visceral innervation.

Includes index.
    1. Nervous system, Autonomic. I. Young, Paul A.,
joint author. II. Biggerstaff, Donald E., joint author.
III. Title. DNLM: 1. Autonomic nervous system.
WL600 B575f
QP368.B45   612'.89   74-30208
ISBN 0-398-03388-9
ISBN 0-398-03390-0 pbk.

This book is dedicated to
our parents
Was Dev and Subdhra Bhagat
Nicholas and Olive Young
Selby and Theda Biggerstaff

PREFACE

THIS ABUNDANTLY ILLUSTRATED BOOK provides a concise exposition of the autonomic nervous system. It is intended to be used as a core text mainly by students. It is not intended to be a reference text for the research worker. The content of the text represents subjects dealing with the anatomy, physiology, and pharmacology of the autonomic nervous system taught to our students in the past two decades. This book should be, therefore, on the desk of every medical student and other persons who want to learn about the anatomy and physiology of the autonomic nervous system.

During the past decade, due to studies in electron microscopy and to the development of specific chemical methods for the identification and measurement of transmitters in tissues, considerable advances have been made in our knowledge of the autonomic nervous system. In preparing this text, an effort has been made to incorporate the results of recent research and newer attitudes and to indicate what appears to be a coming trend. Space limitations prohibit giving references.

We wish to express our appreciation to Mrs. Jo Ann Higdon, Miss Marian F. Parmley, and Mrs. Margaret A. Pomranz for typing the manuscript, and we are especially grateful to Miss Judy Wilson and Miss Ruth Gillies for their secretarial and editorial assistance.

Budh D. Bhagat
Paul A. Young
Donald E. Biggerstaff

CONTENTS

FUNDAMENTALS OF VISCERAL INNERVATION

CHAPTER 1

THE NEURON

O NE OF THE FUNDAMENTAL properties of all animals is the
ability to respond to environmental changes. Such responses in higher animals are mediated by specialized tissue
that forms the nervous system. Basically, nervous tissue has
two main functions: (1) irritability or the capacity to respond
to a stimulus, and (2) conductivity or the capacity to transmit
impulses rapidly over long distances without any loss of signal
strength.

The nervous system of man (and all animals down to the
primitive coelenterates) is composed of individual functional
units, the neurons, which are arranged in chains that form circuits. Each neuron consists of a cell body, one or more protoplasmic processes, called dendrites (if they conduct toward
the cell body) or axons (if they conduct away from the cell
body), and terminals. Neurons are morphologically classified in
terms of their number of cytoplasmic processes. They are unipolar (one process), bipolar (two processes), and multipolar
(three or more processes).

Some special features of neurons are their ectodermal origin,
their inability to reproduce new neurons, their extreme depen-
dence on a constant supply of oxygen and glucose, and the
trophic nature of their cell bodies.

3

Cell Body

The nerve cell is surrounded by a plasma (cell) membrane formed by three lipoprotein layers with an overall thickness of 70 to 80Å. Localized specializations occur at synaptic and adhesive junctions and at the initial segment of the axon.

The nucleus of a nerve cell is within the cell body and is usually centrally located. In many autonomic neurons, however, nuclei are eccentric in location. The nucleus contains dust-like chromatin rich in DNA, and one or more prominent nucleoli, rich in RNA. In neurons of females, a small nucleolar satellite rich in DNA is frequently attached to the periphery of the nucleolus and is thought to represent an X chromosome.

Ultrastructurally, the nucleus is surrounded by a nuclear envelope consisting of two membranes, inner and outer. Each is about 70Å in diameter, and they are separated from each other by a space of varying diameter. The inner membrane is smooth, whereas the outer is ruffled and frequently continuous with the endoplasmic reticulum. The membranes are periodically interrupted by pores which occasionally appear to be closed by a thin membrane. The nucleolus consists of an interwoven mass of granules (pars amorpha) and fine filaments (nucleonema).

Within the cytoplasm of the perikaryon and large dendrites are Nissl bodies consisting of plates or cisterns of rough endoplasmic reticulum and free ribosomes; both are the sites for protein synthesis. These Nissl bodies are absent in the axon hillock. In addition, smooth endoplasmic reticulum known as the Golgi apparatus, is present and is believed to be concerned with secretion of intracellular material such as enzymes and structural macromolecules. Although the Golgi apparatus is usually perinuclear in position, it may extend into the proximal parts of larger dendrites. Mitochondria, which occur throughout the nerve cell body and its processes, present the same morphological features as in other cells. In addition to oxidative phosphorylation, neuronal mitochondria perhaps incorporate amino acids into protein. Thus, the cell body containing the nucleus and many constituents involved in metabolic processes, is responsible for maintaining the metabolism of the neuron including its growth and repair.

Neurofibrils, readily demonstrated by reduced silver methods as elongated structures extending throughout the cytoplasm of the cell body and its processes, are thought to be aggregates of microtubules and neurofilaments. Microtubules, elongated tubular structures from about 200 to 300Å in diameter, are more abundant in dendrites, whereas neurofilaments, tubular structures about 100Å in diameter, are more prevalent in axons. In addition to providing cellular support, the neurofibrils may enhance cytoplasmic flow from the cell body to the distal parts of the neuronal processes. It has been shown that disruption of the neurofilament impairs the axoplasmic flow of many neuronal constituents. Features of the nerve cell body are presented in Figure 1.

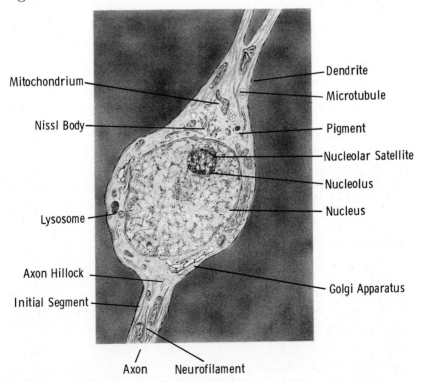

Figure 1. Illustration showing the ultrastructural features of a neuron.

Axons

The axon is the protoplasmic process that carries the nerve impulse away from the cell body. Characteristically they are longer than dendrites and do not taper. Also, axons are covered whereas dendrites are naked. A comparison of axons and dendrites is given in Table I.

TABLE I
COMPARISON OF AXONS AND DENDRITES

Feature	Axon	Dendrite
Length	Longer	Shorter
Diameter	Uniform	Tapers
Branching	Collaterals at right angles	Profuse and at acute angles
Surface	Smooth	Spiny
Coverings	Neurolemma in PNS Myelin in PNS & CNS	Naked
Nissl	None	Present in larger
Ultrastructure	Longitudinal neurofilaments	Longitudinal microtubules
Conduction	Away from soma	Toward soma

The axon emanates from the neuronal soma at the axon hillock. The first part of the axon is called the initial segment. In myelinated axons the initial segment extends as far as the beginning of the myelin sheath. Branches of axons, referred to as collaterals, are few in number and usually arise at right angles to the axon.

The axolemma, or plasma membrane of the axon, has the same characteristics as the unit membrane. It is modified at the initial segment, at nodes of Ranvier, in paranodal regions,. and at synaptic sites.

The axoplasm contains mitochondria, neurofilaments, microtubules, agranular endoplasmic reticulum, and various vesicles. However, it does not contain granular endoplasmic reticulum or ribosomes. In contrast to dendritic cytoplasm, axoplasm contains relatively few microtubules and many neurofilaments. Both of these are oriented parallel to the long axis of the axon. In contrast to both dendrite and cell body, the axon possesses no apparent synthesizing capacity of its own. It is believed that the cell body synthesizes all the necessary macromolecules for the axon, and axoplasmic flow carries them from the cell body to all distal parts of the axon.

Axons may be either myelinated or nonmyelinated. Myelinated axons are surrounded by a sheath of fatty material known as myelin. This layer of lipid material is of variable thickness. The myelin sheath in the central nervous system is formed in the oligodendrocytes, whereas in the peripheral nervous system, it is formed in the Schwann cells. In both cases, it develops by a spiral wrapping of the respective cell around the axon. At intervals varying from 0.2 to 1 mm, the myelin sheath is interrupted by short gaps called the nodes of Ranvier (Fig. 2).

Unmyelinated axons in the peripheral nervous system are located in troughs, or gutters, in Schwann cells. In the brain and spinal cord, they are related to glial elements.

In the peripheral nervous system, individual myelinated and unmyelinated fibers are invested by loosely arranged connective tissue, the *endoneurium*. Groups of these fibers are gathered in variable sized bundles and are surrounded by a dense and lamellated connective tissue sheath, the *perineurium*, which continues to surround the bundles, even after they branch. Groups of bundles are loosely held together by an external connective tissue covering, the *epineurium*. This entire assembly is called a nerve.

Terminals

Interneuronal

Except for unipolar and bipolar nerve cells in the cerebrospinal ganglia, the soma and dendrites of virtually all other neurons have a vast number of terminal endings from axons of other neurons. These junctions between neurons are called synapses and serve to transmit the impulses from one neuron to another. Synapses are dynamically polarized so that the im-

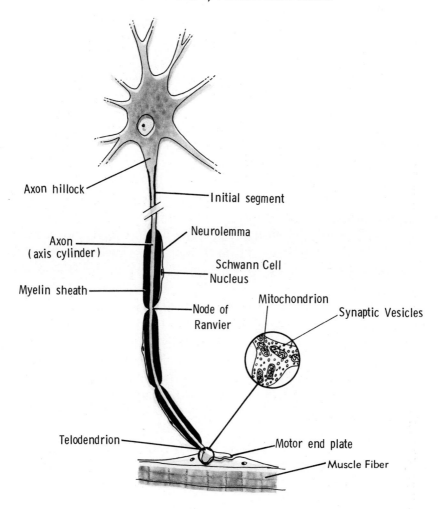

Figure 2. Illustration of motor nerve fiber.

pulses always pass from the terminal ending of the first neuron
to the surface of the second neuron.

With light microscopy the terminal axons exhibit a wide
variety of forms, the most common being round end-loops called
boutons. Electron microscopy has revealed that the axon terminal, or bouton, is filled with large numbers of membrane-
bound vesicles and numerous mitochondria.

The synaptic surface of the bouton possesses a distinct pre-synaptic membrane which is separated from the postsynaptic part of the target neuron by a gap, or synaptic cleft. Variations in the width of the synaptic cleft characterize synapses as either electrical or chemical (see Fig. 4 below.) Electrically coupled synapses commonly show fusion of the pre- and post-synaptic membranes. Chemically coupled synapses possess gaps that measure between 200 to 600Å. During the process of chemical transmission, an electrical signal in the presynaptic membrane causes the release of a transmitter into the synaptic cleft where it interacts with a specific site (called a receptor) on the postsynaptic membrane to initiate an action potential.

Neuromuscular

The terminal parts of motor axons assume specialized forms where they synapse on skeletal or smooth muscle.

In the case of the somatic system, the motor axon loses its my-elin sheath and divides into numerous branches immediately before it reaches the muscle fibers to be innervated (Fig. 3). A single axon may innervate hundreds of muscle fibers. The alpha motor neuron, its axon, and the muscle fibers it innervates is a motor unit. The size of motor units varies tremendously, since a single somatic motor axon may supply from twenty or thirty to over a thousand or more muscle fibers.

The region of the muscle fiber which makes contact with the motor nerve is called a motor end-plate (Fig. 5). The axon terminal is discretely isolated from the surface of the muscle by a synaptic cleft.

Terminals of autonomic axons on smooth muscle are far more complex and differ from somatic motor terminals in the following ways:

1. the autonomic terminal axon becomes varicose as it ap-proaches the effector cell, whereas the somatic axon does not;

2. relatively few of all the fibers of a smooth muscle bundle receive a terminal twig, whereas every skeletal muscle fiber has a motor end-plate;

3. the autonomic terminal axon is within a bundle con-

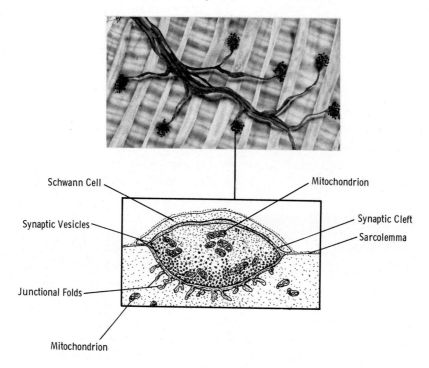

Figure 3. Illustration and schematic drawing of a myoneural junction. Motor nerve fiber within a nerve trunk originates from an alpha motor neuron. Just before it reaches the muscle it innervates, the axon loses its myelin sheath and divides into a number of branches. Each branch terminates on a single muscle fiber. The region of the muscle fiber with which the nerve makes contact is known as the end-plate. An alpha motor neuron and the muscle fibers it innervates is a motor unit.

taining terminals from many axons. Thus, a smooth muscle fiber may be innervated by terminals of different axons, whereas a somatic muscle fiber is innervated by only one axon.

A feature of all chemical nerve terminals both interneuronal and neuromuscular, is the presence of intracellular synaptic vesicles. These vesicles measure from 200 to 800Å in diameter. Some have an electron-dense core while others have an electron-translucent core. These vesicles are the storage sites for chemical substances.

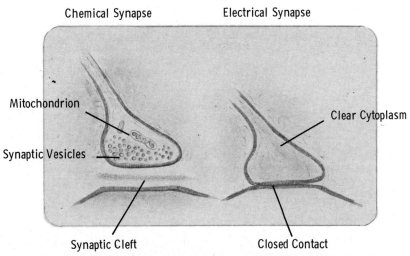

Chemical Synapse   Electrical Synapse

Mitochondrion

Synaptic Vesicles

Clear Cytoplasm

Synaptic Cleft   Closed Contact

Figure 4. Schematic representation of chemical and electrical synapses. In a chemical synapse, the postsynaptic membrane is separated by a synaptic cleft. The presynaptic site has vesicles containing transmitter. In an electrical synapse, pre- and post-synaptic membranes are fused.

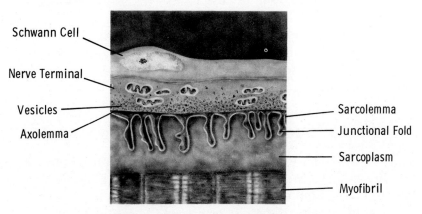

Schwann Cell

Nerve Terminal

Vesicles

Axolemma

Sarcolemma

Junctional Fold

Sarcoplasm

Myofibril

Figure 5. Illustration of motor end-plate ultrastructure.

AXOPLASMIC TRANSPORT

The cell body of a neuron is the trophic center of the entire cell. Because of the astronomical distance between the perikaryon and the axon terminals of a neuron, a special mechanism called axoplasmic transport conveys metabolic materials from one part of the cell to another.

There is ample evidence that the enzymes necessary for the synthesis of neurotransmitters and the protein components of the vesicles are synthesized in the cell body and transported to the terminals by axoplasmic flow. Thus, when a postganglionic sympathetic axon is ligated, endogenous norepinephrine with its granular vesicles and enzymes such as dopamine β hydroxylase accumulate proximal to, but not distal to, the ligature. Also, when two ligatures are placed on the same axon, no accumulation of transported materials occurs proximal to the more distal ligature. These observations confirm the proximo-distal direction of the transport.

Axoplasmic transport is a highly specialized phenomenon and the various axoplasmic constituents are transported at varying rates. Some protein components such as vesicles and mitochondria are transported rapidly (5–6 mm/hour), whereas others flow more slowly (1 mm/day).

The exact mechanism of axoplasmic transport is unknown. The microtubules have been implicated in the rapid transport of vesicles and mitochondria. Thus, mitotic inhibitors such as colchicine and vinblastine, which cause disruption of microtubules, block the somatofugal transport of norepinephrine and dense core vesicles in sympathetic neurons.

BIOELECTRIC PROPERTIES OF NERVE FIBERS

The function of an axon is to transmit impulses from one neuron to another. In order to perform this function the axon propagates an impulse along its length.

When the electrical activity of an axon is recorded at various points on the surface of its resting membrane or axolemma, there is no difference in potential from one point to another, that is, all the points on the surface are isopotential. In contrast, when electrical activity is recorded on the surface of and deep to the axolemma (transmembrane), there is always a difference in the potential, the inside being -70 to -90 mv as compared to the outside. This difference in electrical potential is known as the *resting* or *polarized potential.* Thus, in a normal resting condition the axon exhibits a steady difference of electrical potential across its membrane.

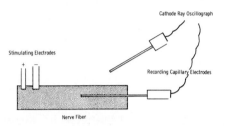

Figure 6 A. Shows the method of measuring resting and action potentials. Fine glass capillary tubes filled with saturated KCl solution are inserted into the axoplasm. This forms the inner electrode. One outward electrode is also KCl.

When an axon is stimulated, the transmembrane potential is reversed for a short while, that is, the inside of the membrane becomes positive with respect to the outside. The size of this overshoot is 30 to 50 mv (Fig. 6, A, B.) This reversal of potential initiates a nerve impulse and is known as the *action potential.*

The action potential follows the *all or none law,* according to which the action potential is produced only when the intensity of the stimulus reaches a certain critical level known as the *threshold level.* Any stimulus weaker than this, is a *subthreshold stimulus* and will not trigger an action potential. Stimulus intensities above the threshold level do not alter the magnitude, shape, or duration of the action potential. That is, a *suprathreshold stimulus* will produce an action potential identical to that produced by a threshold stimulus. The threshold of stimulation is inversely proportional to the diameter of the nerve fiber, thus, large myelinated fibers usually have higher thresholds of stimulation.

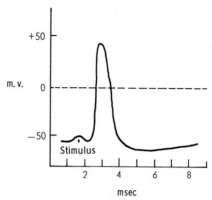

Figure 6 B. Action potential.

A nerve trunk consists of hundreds of nerve fibers whose thresholds are spread over a wide range. When the stimulus strength is increased above the threshold, it causes excitation of more and more fibers and the twitch increases in strength. When the point is reached where the strength of the impulse ceases to increase further, it is assumed that all the fibers in the nerve trunk are being triggered; this requires a *maximal stimulus.*

Refractory Period

Shortly after a stimulus initiates an impulse, the nerve enters a refractory state for one or two milliseconds. During this period, it is impossible to initiate a second impulse. This is called the *absolute refractory period* and is followed by a relative refractory period during which a suprathreshold stimulus is required to set up an impulse. However, the amplitude of such a response is smaller than the normal response. Thus, it is possible to determine the degree of recovery of an axon by measuring the amplitude of the second stimulus. Usually the absolute refractory period for mammalian axons is about 0.5 msec.

Propagation of the Nerve Impulse

On stimulation, the stimulated point of the membrane becomes negatively charged with respect to the adjacent point which is normally positively charged. A local current is set up between the resting and active points (Fig. 7A). This local current acts as the stimulus resulting in a depolarization of the adjacent resting point and its potential reverses from positive to negative. The action point thus has shifted from the originally stimulated point to the adjacent point on the membrane. In this way, the action potential travels, point by point, along the nerve fiber.

Thus, the propagation of an impulse depends essentially on the flow of current in a local circuit ahead of the active region which depolarizes the resting membrane and causes it in turn to become active.

When the action potential has shifted from one point on the membrane to the next, the first point becomes repolarized, i.e. its resting potential has recovered.

Saltatory Conduction

Since the myelin sheath is a good insulator the electrical resistance of the axolemma along the internodal portion of the nerve fiber is greatly increased. A stimulating current which generates the action potential has its effect at the node of Ranvier. Due to the insulation of the myelin sheath, the local current produced at one node of Ranvier cannot pass through the internodal region of the axon membrane. The current propagates in the axoplasm and at the adjacent node it passes back into the extracellular fluid. Thus, there is activation in a node to node succession without any contribution from the long internodal zone (Fig. 7B). As a result, the activity in the myelinated fiber jumps (about a mm at a jump) from node to node in contrast to the continuous wave-like progression in a nonmyelinated fiber. This conduction in the myelinated fiber is known as *saltatory conduction*.

As a consequence of the current flow being restricted to the nodal region, the conduction velocity is many times greater than that in a nonmyelinated fiber of the same diameter, and there is a great economy in the energy expenditure because only

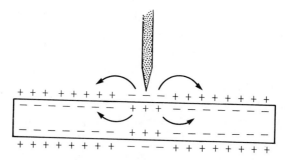

Figure 7 A. Shows the local circuit theory in the non myelinated fiber.

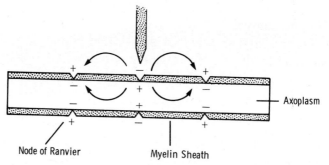

Figure 7 B. Shows the saltatory conduction in a myelinated nerve fiber.

a fraction of the axon membrane presumably undergoes de-polarization during activity.

Membrane Theory of Nervous Conduction

A plasma membrane of 50 to 100 Å thickness surrounds the cytoplasm of nerve and muscle cells. It separates the internal aqueous protoplasm from the extracellular fluid. Both aqueous solutions have a very different ionic composition. The extra-cellular fluid has a high concentration of sodium and chloride ions and is relatively low in potassium ion concentration. Within the cell, sodium and chloride ions are at a lower concentration than on the outside. Potassium ions are about twenty to fifty times more concentrated within the cell than they are outside the cell. The bulk of the internal ions consist of organic mole-cules, mainly amino acids. Sodium and potassium ions carry positive charges whereas chloride ions have a negative charge. The organic ions within the cell are negatively charged. The separation of these electrically charged particles by the plasma membrane sets up a potential difference across the membrane, so that the interior of the resting membrane is about 70 to 80 mv negative with respect to the exterior.

Equilibrium Potential

The mobilities of the ions across the membrane differ and may be influenced by at least three factors:

1. *The permeability of the membrane to the ions.* The membrane acts as a physical restraint on the diffusion of ions. The membrane is relatively more permeable to potassium and chloride ions than to sodium ions. Organic ions cannot leave the cell by diffusion because of their large size.
2. *The concentration gradient.* Because of the unequal distribution of the ions across the membrane, ions will tend to diffuse from regions where their concentration is high to regions where it is low.
3. *The electrical gradient.* Ions which are charged positively will tend to diffuse towards the regions of negative charge and vice versa.

Potassium can flow back and forth across the membrane with relative ease. It has a higher concentration inside the cell than outside. According to the concentration gradient, potassium should diffuse out of the cell. Since potassium carries a positive charge, as it diffuses out it creates greater and greater negativity within the cell. The resulting membrane potential opposes the further movement of potassium ions. Thus, as the potassium ions diffuse out, the concentration gradient decreases whereas the membrane potential increases since both opposing forces are equal. At this stage potassium ions move at equal rates in both directions. The membrane potential that just stops net diffusion of ions across the membrane is called its equilibrium potential. Equilibrium potentials are denoted by E. Nernst made a study of equilibria of this sort and derived an equation to describe them. Using this equation the potential difference can be calculated, provided the concentration of ions is known.

The Nernst formula is

$$E = K \log \frac{(\text{ionic concentration on one side})}{(\text{ionic concentration on the other side})}$$

where E is the equilibrium potential, K is a constant and depends among other things upon absolute temperature.

The inside of the cell is negative in reference to the outside. Therefore, the electrical gradient is inward for positive ions and outward for negative ions. In the case of potassium the electrical gradient is inward. The calculated equilibrium potential however is higher (—96 mv) than the actual membrane potential (— 70 mv). This means that the potassium concentration within the cell is more than is accounted for by the electrochemical gradient. There must be an additional force which is responsible for pumping the potassium within the cell against the electrochemical gradient. This concept of an active pump is supported by the fact that the potassium ion influx measured with radioactive potassium is reduced by poisoning the pump with ouabain.

The equilibrium potential for sodium is + 60 mv. Both the concentration gradient and the electrical gradient are inward yet there is far more sodium outside the cell than within the cell.

Hodgkin and his co-workers pushed a fine glass capillary tube into a squid axon and injected a small quantity of radioactive sodium. Within a few seconds, radioactivity began to appear in the extracellular fluid bathing the fiber. This indicates that the membrane is not completely impermeable to sodium ions.

To explain the concentration of sodium ions within the cell, it has been suggested that a metabolic pump exists in the membrane. This pump drives sodium ions from the inside of the cell to the outside against a high concentration and electrical gradient (which tend to force it in) and thereby maintains a relatively low intracellular concentration of sodium. This pump uses metabolic energy from adenosine triphosphate (ATP) hydroly-sis. Metabolic poisons such as dinitrophenol and ouabain can block it. These drugs stop the pump by interfering with the utilization of ATP.

The sodium and potassium pumps may be loosely coupled together and driven by the same metabolic process which moves the two ions simultaneously. It has been shown that inward movement of sodium ions is linked with the outward movement of potassium ions; for every three sodium ions pumped out there are two potassium ions transported into the cell. Thus, the sodium/potassium pump is responsible for maintaining the ionic imbalance. This imbalance of electrically charged particles makes possible the establishment of a potential difference across the membrane.

Hodgkin and his co-workers have shown that sodium con-ductance (rate of diffusion across the membrane) is a function of the membrane potential. When the membrane is at the rest-ing potential sodium conductance is very low; it increases smoothly as the membrane is depolarized.

When a nerve is stimulated, the decrease in the membrane potential leads to an increase in sodium conductance. Sodium ions begin to flow into the cell along its electrical and concentra-tion gradient. If the initial depolarization is large enough, sodium ions enter faster than the potassium efflux; this leads to a very rapid rise of the action potential because sodium ions carry into the cell the positive charge and reduce the internal negativity. Thus, as the sodium ions flow in, the membrane becomes more and more depolarized. This influx of sodium ions further increases the permeability to sodium (Fig. 8). The entry of sodium ions could continue until sodium ions approach their equilibrium potential which is about + 60 mv. However, the peak of the action potential does not reach the equilibrium po-tential of sodium since a marked increase in sodium conductance is of short duration. The mechanism of automatic inactivation of sodium membrane permeability is not fully known, but in-activation of sodium membrane permeability is an important factor in the termination of the action potential. Local anesthetics block activation of the sodium conductance preventing depolarization.

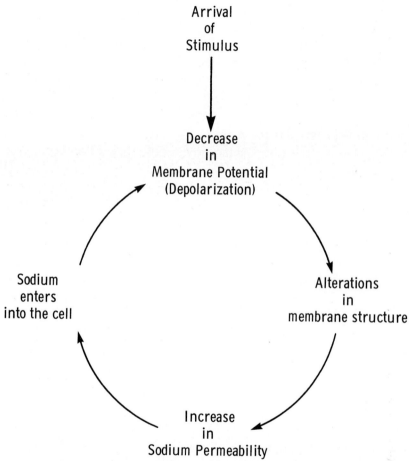

Figure 8. Diagram showing the linkage between membrane depolarization and increased sodium permeability.

While the influx of sodium ions is taking place during the action potential, the membrane becomes temporarily impermeable to potassium. As the sodium permeability declines, the potassium permeability rises and potassium ions begin to leave the fiber. This efflux of potassium continues until the inside of the fiber is sufficiently negative with respect to the outside to prevent potassium ions leaving, i.e. until potassium ions reach their equilibrium potential. The membrane becomes repolarized. Thus the rising phase and peak of the action potential are due to a large but transient rise in sodium conductance, whereas the falling phase of the action potential is due to inactivation of the sodium permeability changes and to an outward movement of potassium ions. Sodium conductance starts at an exceedingly low value but rises rapidly and then declines exponentially. The potassium conductance is generated slowly but rises in a S-shaped curve to a steady level.

On the basis of the sodium ion hypothesis, the threshold is the potential at which sodium influx balances the outward potassium current. For *subthreshold* depolarization the inward sodium current is not strong enough to balance the outward potassium current, and the membrane repolarizes to its resting value. At a critical potential the sodium influx equals the potassium efflux. The potential lingers for some time in a state of unstable equilibrium. It may turn upward into an action potential or it may turn downward to a resting level.

At the end of the spike, both sodium conductance and potassium conductance are greater than the resting and, as a result, the threshold for reexcitation is raised. Until the permeabilities for both ions return to normal values, a greater stimulus (above the normal threshold) is necessary to trigger a second spike. This explains why there is a refractory period before a second impulse can be triggered. When an impulse has passed along an axon, there is little change in ion concentration, very little sodium has been gained, and little potassium is lost. Actually it is the permeability of the nerve membrane which alters during action potential, not the concentration of the ions within the cell.

CHAPTER 2

ANATOMY OF THE VISCERAL MOTOR SYSTEM

Subdivision of the Nervous System

THE NERVOUS SYSTEM is conceptually subdivided into central and peripheral parts (Table II). The central nervous system includes the brain and spinal cord, whereas the peripheral includes the cerebrospinal and autonomic nerves and ganglia. It must be emphasized that these divisions are solely for descriptive purposes since neither anatomically nor physiologically is any one part of the nervous system independent of the other.

The autonomic system innervates visceral organs including the vascular and glandular systems. Since it generally acts below the level of consciousness, it is involuntary and functions to maintain homeostasis of the internal environment, e.g. body temperature, blood pressure.

Functionally, the autonomic system consists of all central and peripheral nerve cells and fibers that influence visceral activity. Thus the afferent and efferent visceral nerves, as well as the central autonomic paths, should be included. By traditional definition, however, the autonomic system is purely efferent. In view of their functional importance, the visceral afferent fibers and central autonomic pathways, although not included in this system by traditional definition, will be considered.

TABLE II

DIVISIONS OF NERVOUS SYSTEM

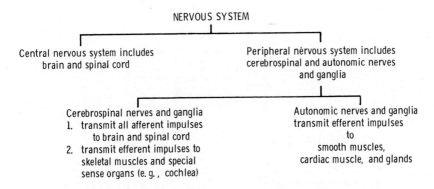

NERVOUS SYSTEM	
Central nervous system includes brain and spinal cord	Peripheral nervous system includes cerebrospinal and autonomic nerves and ganglia
Cerebrospinal nerves and ganglia 1. transmit all afferent impulses to brain and spinal cord 2. transmit efferent impulses to skeletal muscles and special sense organs (e. g. , cochlea)	Autonomic nerves and ganglia transmit efferent impulses to smooth muscles, cardiac muscle, and glands

Comparison of Visceral and Somatic Motor Systems

Although components of the visceral and somatic systems intermingle and overlap both centrally and peripherally, few similarities exist between the two systems. For example, even the basic spinal reflex arcs differ.

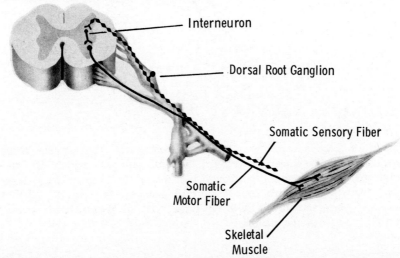

Figure 9. Schematic representation of simple somatic reflex arc. The reflex consists of a) somatic sensory fiber with its cell body in the spinal ganglion, b) interneuron in the spinal cord, and c) alpha motor neuron with its somatic motor fiber going to skeletal muscle.

FIGURE 10A

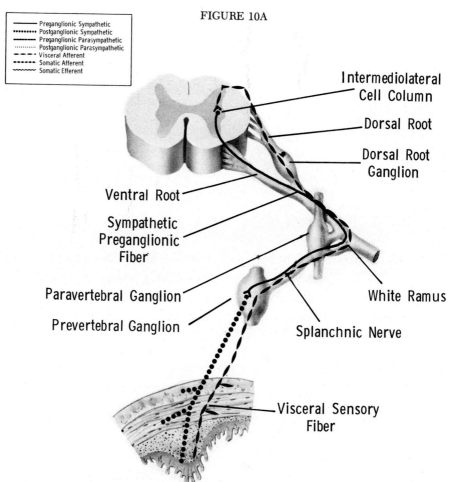

Preganglionic Sympathetic
Postganglionic Sympathetic
Preganglionic Parasympathetic
Postganglionic Parasympathetic
Visceral Afferent
Somatic Afferent
Somatic Efferent

Intermediolateral
Cell Column

Dorsal Root

Dorsal Root
Ganglion

Ventral Root

Sympathetic
Preganglionic
Fiber

Paravertebral Ganglion

Prevertebral Ganglion

White Ramus

Splanchnic Nerve

Visceral Sensory
Fiber

Figure 10. Illustrations of simple visceral reflex arcs. The simplest reflex would consist of three neurons: a) visceral afferent neuron, b) preganglionic neuron, and c) postganglionic neuron. It is more likely, however, that these reflexes consist of four neurons: a) visceral afferent neuron, b) an interneuron within the spinal cord, c) preganglionic neuron, and d) postganglionic neuron.

Simple spinal somatic reflex arcs (Fig. 9) most commonly involve three neurons:

1. *Afferent neuron.* The cell body is a unipolar dorsal root

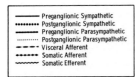

FIGURE 10B

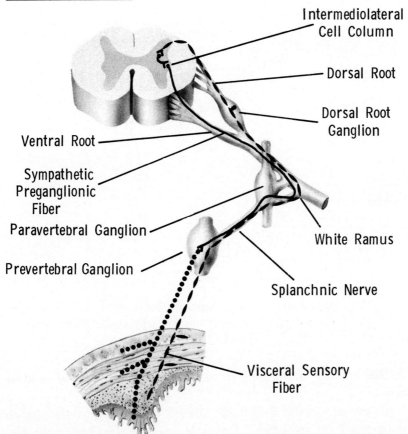

ganglion cell. Its axon terminates peripherally in the skin or some other somatic tissue usually as a receptor associated with pain. The central branch terminates in the posterior horn of the spinal cord.

2. *Interneuron.* The cell body is located in the posterior horn and its axon transmits impulses to cells in the anterior horn. All parts of this neuron are in the spinal gray matter.

3. *Efferent neuron.* This is an alpha motor neuron located

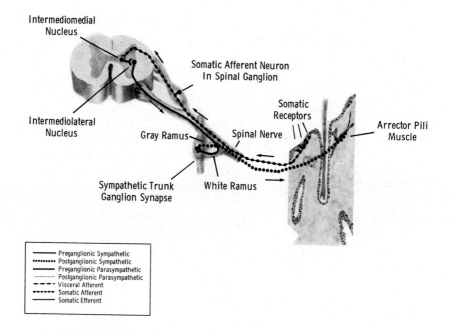

Figure 11. Illustration of simple somato-visceral reflex arc. The reflex consists of four neurons: a) somatic afferent neuron, b) interneuron, c) preganglionic neuron, and d) postganglionic neuron.

in the anterior horn and its axon innervates skeletal muscle fibers.

A simpler somatic reflex, the stretch or myotatic reflex which is initiated by stretching a muscle spindle, involves only two neurons since the afferent neuron synapses directly on the efferent neuron.

Usually, the simplest spinal visceral reflex arc involves four neurons (Fig. 10b):

1. *Afferent neuron.* The cell body is unipolar and located in a dorsal root ganglion. Peripherally its axon terminates in a visceral receptor located in the wall of an organ or blood vessel; centrally it synapses on an interneuron in the spinal cord.

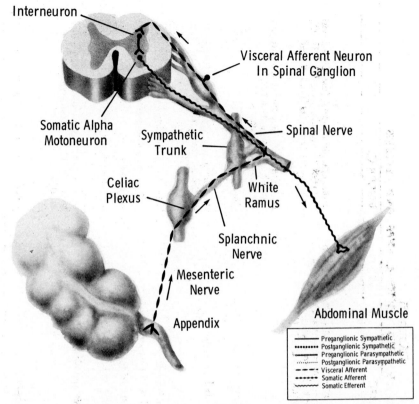

Figure 12. Illustration of simple viscero-somatic reflex arc. The reflex consists of three neurons: a) visceral afferent neuron, b) interneuron, and c) somatic efferent neuron.

2. *Interneuron.* This neuron is located in the intermediate zone and its axon transmits impulses to neurons in the lateral horn. All parts of this neuron are in the spinal gray matter.

3. *Preganglionic neuron.* Located in the lateral horn, this neuron has an axon which passes from the spinal cord and synapses in an autonomic ganglion.

4. *Postganglionic neuron.* This neuron is located in an autonomic ganglion and its axon innervates smooth muscle or cardiac muscle or gland cells.

The attempts by earlier authors to describe similarities between the basic components of somatic and visceral reflex arcs

TABLE III
COMPARISON OF SOMATIC AND VISCERAL EFFERENT SYSTEMS

PARTS	SOMATIC	VISCERAL
1. Nervous Parts		
A. Central neurons	Alpha motor neurons (associated with nuclei of all cerebrospinal nerves except olfactory, optic, and vestibulocochlear)	Preganglionic neurons (associated with nuclei of cranial nerves III, VII, IX, X, spinal segments T.1-L.2, and S.2-4)
B. Peripheral neurons	None	Postganglionic neurons in sympathetic trunk, autonomic plexus, and terminal ganglia
C. Pathway from CNS to effector	Uninterrupted	One synapse
D. Fiber types	Myelinated (A type)	Preganglionic: Myelinated (B type) Postganglionic: Unmyelinated (C type)
2. Effector Parts		
A. Types	Skeletal muscle	Smooth and cardiac muscles; glands
B. Influenced by	Central nervous system only	Central or peripheral nervous system
C. Initiation of activity	Voluntary or reflex	Reflex only
D. Responses to stimulation	Excitation only	Either excitation or inhibition
E. Responses to denervation	Paralysis and atrophy	Dysfunction varies with organ; usually little change in automaticity and no atrophy
3. Chemical Parts		
A. Neurotransmitter	Acetylcholine	Acetylcholine and norepinephrine

were based on the theory that both consisted of three neurons. In this case the somatic interneuron was equated to the autonomic preganglionic neuron (Fig. 10a). However, recent evidence shows an absence of dorsal root fibers terminating in the lateral zone. This indicates that an interneuron exists between the visceral afferent and the preganglionic neuron (Fig. 10b).

Reflexes involving somatic and visceral nerves also exist. Examples of simple somato-visceral and viscero-somatic reflexes are illustrated in Figures 11 and 12 .

In addition to differences in the basic reflexes, there are other important anatomical and physiological differences between the somatic and visceral efferent systems. These differences are summarized in Table III.

General Features of Visceral Innervation

The autonomic system has two major parts: the sympathetic (orthosympathetic) and the parasympathetic. The efferent paths, whether motor or secretory, consist of two neuron circuits from the brain or spinal cord to the effector organ. The proximal or preganglionic components have their cell bodies in the brain or spinal cord and their axons synapse in the autonomic ganglia of the peripheral nervous system. The distal or postganglionic components are entirely in the peripheral nervous system; their cell bodies are in the autonomic ganglia and their axons innervate smooth muscle, cardiac muscle, and exocrine glands.

Preganglionic Components (Figs. 13 and 14)

The cell bodies of preganglionic sympathetic neurons are located in the twelve thoracic and upper two lumbar spinal cord segments. Those of the parasympathetic system are in the midbrain, pontine, and medullary regions of the brain stem and in the second, third, and fourth sacral segments of the spinal cord. Hence, in reference to the locations of preganglionic cell bodies, synonymous terms for sympathetic and parasympathetic are thoracolumbar and craniosacral respectively.

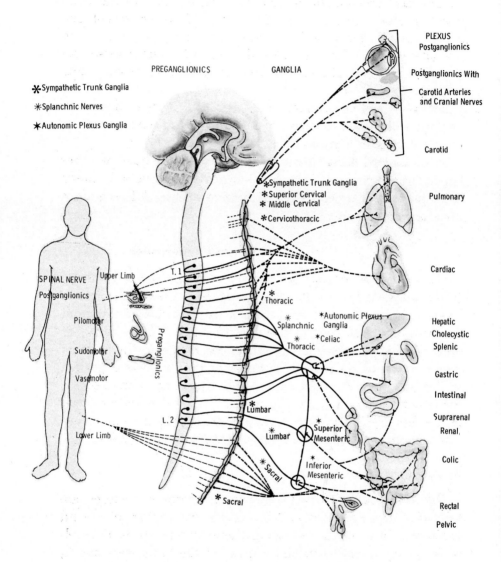

Figure 13. Schematic representation of sympathetic system

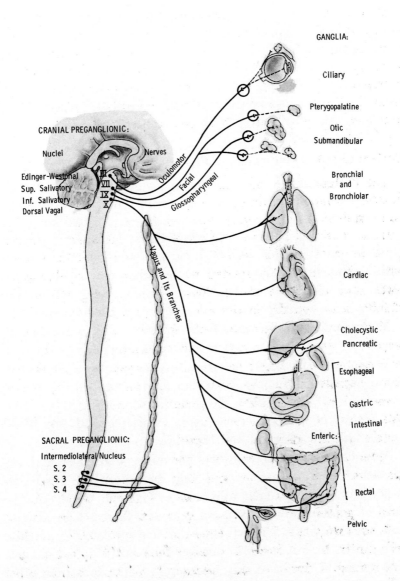

Figure 14. Schematic representation of parasympathetic system

Microscopically, the preganglionic neurons within the brain stem and spinal cord are small or medium-sized multipolar cells with highly variable shapes. A slim cytoplasmic margin with small Nissl bodies surrounds the large nucleus which contains a prominent nucleolus (Fig. 1). The preganglionic axons emerge from the brain or spinal cord as small myelinated type-B fibers and pass via peripheral nerves to autonomic ganglia.

Postganglionic Components (Figs. 13 and 14)

The postganglionic neurons are in ganglia located at various distances from the central nervous system. Thus, there are: (1) paravertebral ganglia within the sympathetic trunks lying beside the vertebral column, (2) prevertebral (collateral) ganglia lying in front of the vertebral column and actually located within plexuses closely related to branches of the abdominal aorta, and (3) terminal (intrinsic) ganglia lying within the vicinity of or actually in the effector organs themselves.

Microscopically, the autonomic ganglia vary somewhat in respect to size, shape, number, and arrangement of postganglionic neurons. The larger ganglia are enclosed by a connective tissue capsule continuous with the epineurium of the nerves connected with it. Within the ganglia, supporting tissue consists mainly of the connective tissue associated with the blood vessels and the ganglion cell capsules.

Autonomic ganglion cells are generally multipolar and are characterized by numerous and long dendrites. The Nissl substance has a fine granular appearance. Pigment, usually in the form of golden brown lipofuscin granules, increases in amount with advancing age. The cell bodies are encapsulated by satellite cells similar to, but fewer in number than in the spinal ganglia. The numerous dendrites may intermingle with axons from other cells either internal or external to the capsule. The postganglionic axon is usually of the unmyelinated type-C. The terminal ganglia within walls of visceral organs consist of small groups of multipolar neurons intermingled with dendrites and axons.

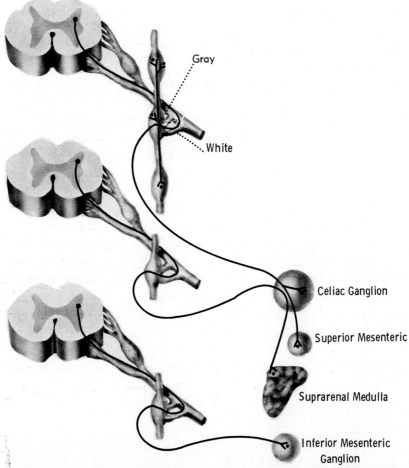

Gray

White

Celiac Ganglion

Superior Mesenteric

Suprarenal Medulla

Inferior Mesenteric
Ganglion

Figure 15. Schematic representation of connections of sympathetic preganglionic fibers. Preganglionic fibers originate from the intermediolateral
cell column of spinal cord segments T.1 to L.2. They reach adjacent
sympathetic trunk ganglia where they may synapse or pass through. Some
ascend to synapse in ganglia higher up, and some descend to synapse in
ganglia lower down; others emerge to end in the autonomic plexus ganglia
or the suprarenal medulla.

Sympathetic Nerves

Preganglionic Parts (Fig. 15)

Cell bodies of sympathetic preganglionic neurons are found

solely in the thoracic and upper lumbar segments of the spinal cord. These "thoracolumbar components" form the intermediolateral cell column located in the lateral horn of spinal cord segments T.1 through L.2. The preganglionic axons from these cells emerge in the ventral roots, enter the spinal nerves and course distally in the ventral rami (Fig. 15). At a short distance beyond the intervertebral foramen, each ventral ramus becomes an intercostal or a subcostal nerve and while crossing the posterior aspect of the sympathetic trunk, the nerve communicates with the trunk by means of a white ramus (white because its fibers are myelinated) (Fig. 15). Since sympathetic preganglionic fibers are limited solely to spinal nerves T.1 through L.2, only these nerves possess the white communicating rami.

Upon entering the sympathetic trunk the preganglionic fibers branch in such a manner that one preganglionic fiber may synapse on large numbers of cells either within a single ganglion or several ganglia. The ratio of preganglionic to postganglionic fibers is highly variable and, on the basis of counts, has frequently been estimated to be about 1 : 11 or 12, although counts have gone as high as 1 : 32. This ratio provides the anatomic substrate for the generalized or widespread character of sympathetic reactions.

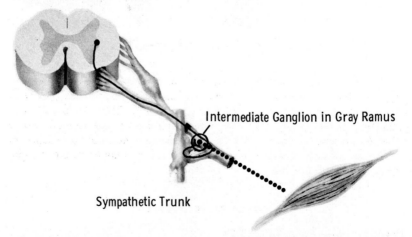

Intermediate Ganglion in Gray Ramus

Sympathetic Trunk

Figure 16. Schematic representation of intermediate ganglion. Some preganglionic sympathetic fibers synapse in intermediate ganglia.

Postganglionic Parts (Fig. 13)

In contrast to the type-B preganglionic fibers, post-ganglionic sympathetic fibers are unmyelinated type-C fibers and have their cells of origin in the ganglia of the sympathetic trunks or in the ganglia lying near certain branches of the abdominal aorta. A variable number of postganglionic sympathetic fibers arise from accessory ganglion cells which migrate during development into communicating rami, spinal nerves, splanchnic nerves, nerves to specific viscera, and even into the walls of various organs (Fig. 16).

Ganglia

Anatomically, sympathetic ganglia are divided into two classes: sympathetic trunk (or paravertebral ganglia) and autonomic plexus (or prevertebral ganglia).

1. *Sympathetic trunk ganglia.* The right and left sympathetic trunks extend from the base of the cranium to the coccyx on the ventrolateral aspects of the vertebral column. Each trunk consists of a series of between twenty to twenty-five ganglia connected by trunk fibers.

In early development, paired primordial ganglia arise from the neural crests of each spinal cord segment. Because of fusions, however, the mature sympathetic trunk contains a variable number of ganglia; usually they number twenty-two or twenty-three (3 cervical, 10–11 thoracic, 4 lumbar, 4 sacral, 1 impar).

A. *Input.* The sympathetic trunks receive their preganglionic fibers via the white communicating rami of spinal nerves T.1 through L.2. Once within the sympathetic trunk, the preganglionic fibers take variable courses (Fig. 15). Some synapse immediately in the trunk ganglia, others ascend or descend to synapse more cranially or caudally in the trunk ganglia, and some pass through the trunk without synapsing to course via the splanchnic nerves to ganglia in the autonomic plexuses.

Preganglionic fibers from spinal segments T.1 to 9 synapse in trunk ganglia at the same or higher levels (Fig. 13). Those from T.5 to 9 may also leave the trunk via the greater splanchnic nerve to synapse in the celiac ganglion.

Preganglionic fibers from spinal segments T.10 through L.2 may synapse in trunk ganglia at the same and lower levels or in the autonomic plexus ganglia after coursing from the sympathetic trunk into the splanchnic nerves.

B. *Output.* The sympathetic trunk ganglion cells supply postganglionic fibers to all the sympathetically-innervated tissues and organs of the body except those in the abdomen, pelvis, and perineum.

Postganglionic fibers from the sympathetic trunk ganglia can be classified according to their courses into perivascular, spinal, and visceral. The perivascular fibers arise mainly in the superior cervical ganglia and course along the carotid arteries to innervate structures in the head. The spinal fibers arise from all trunk ganglia and join each spinal nerve via the gray communicating rami (gray due to unmyelinated fibers). These vasomotor,

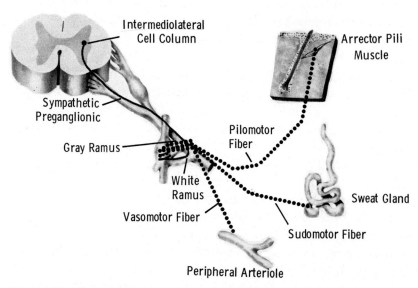

Figure 17. Illustration of neural pathway to peripheral structures. Preganglionic sympathetic fibers synapse in the trunk ganglia, and postganglionic fibers originating there enter all spinal nerves through the gray communicating rami. These vasomotor, sudomotor and pilomotor fibers are solely sympathetic.

sudomotor, and pilomotor fibers are distributed to the upper and lower limbs and the thoracic and abdominal walls (Fig. 17). Visceral fibers in the cervical and thoracic cardiac nerves arise from the cervical and upper thoracic ganglia and pass to the heart and lungs via the cardiac and pulmonary nerves and plexuses. Also, visceral fibers from the lower lumbar ganglia travel in the lumbar splanchnic nerves to the superior hypogastric plexus and those from the sacral ganglia pass to the inferior hypogastric plexus via the sacral splanchnic nerves.

2. *Autonomic plexus ganglia.* Sympathetic innervation of the abdominal, pelvic, and perineal organs mainly involves postganglionic neurons located anterior to the abdominal aorta and closely related to the origins of the celiac, superior mesenteric, and inferior mesenteric arteries (Fig. 13). The celiac ganglia lie at the origin of the celiac trunk, each on a corresponding crus of the diaphragm. Inferolateral extensions of these ganglia, lying at the origins of the renal arteries, are called the aorticorenal ganglia. The superior and inferior mesenteric ganglia, both of which may be single or paired, lie either in front of or on the sides of the respective arteries at their origins.

A. *Input.* The autonomic plexus ganglia receive preganglionic sympathetic fibers whose cells of origin are located in the intermediolateral cell column at spinal cord levels T.5 through L.2. These preganglionic fibers course via their respective ventral roots, spinal nerves, ventral rami, and white communicating rami to the sympathetic trunk, through which they pass without synapsing to emerge in the splanchnic nerves (Fig. 15).

The greater splanchnic nerve carries preganglionic fibers from spinal segments T.5 through 10 and takes origin from a number of large and small roots that emerge from the sympathetic trunk between its fifth and tenth ganglia. After coursing obliquely downward and forward toward the aorta, the roots unite and enter the celiac plexus after piercing the diaphragm or its aortic opening.

The lesser splanchnic nerve, when present, contains preganglionic fibers from spinal segments T.11 through 12 and its roots usually arise from the level of the lower thoracic trunk

TABLE IV

EFFERENT COMPONENTS OF SPLANCHNIC NERVES

Nerve	Origin of Preganglionic Fibers from Spinal Cord Segments	Origin of Postganglionic Fibers from Trunk Ganglia	Attachment of Roots to Sympathetic Trunk	Destination
Greater Splanchnic	T.5–10	—	T5(6)–9(10)	Celiac Plexus
Lesser Splanchnic	T.11–12	—	T 9 & 10 or T 10 & 11	Celiac Plexus
Lowest Splanchnic	T.12	—	T 11	Renal Plexus
Lumbar Splanchnics	L.1–2	—	L 1	Celiac, Renal and Intermesenteric Plexuses
	L.1–2 L.1–2	L3–4 ganglia	L 2 L(2)3(4)	Intermesenteric Plexus Intermesenteric and Superior Hypogastric Plexuses
	L.1–2	L3–4 ganglia	L 4	Superior Hypogastric Plexus
Sacral Splanchnics	L.1–2	S1–4 ganglia	S 1–4	Inferior Hypogastric Plexus
Pelvic Splanchnics (Parasympathetic)	S.2–4	—	—	Inferior Hypogastric Plexus

ganglia. After coursing lateral to the greater splanchnic, the nerve pierces the diaphragm and passes to the celiac and adjacent plexuses. The lowest splanchnic nerve, when present, carries preganglionic fibers from T.12, arises at the level of the lowest thoracic trunk ganglion, enters the abdomen medial to the sympathetic trunk, and joins the renal plexus.

A variable number of lumbar splanchnic nerves (usually 4) carry preganglionic fibers from spinal segments L.1 to 2 and arise from the sympathetic trunk at the levels of the lumbar ganglia. The upper ones pass to the celiac and adjacent plexuses, the middle to the intermesenteric plexus which extends along the aorta between the origins of the superior and inferior mesenteric arteries, and the lower ones pass to the superior hypogastric plexus. The efferent components of the splanchnic nerves are summarized in Table IV.

B. *Output.* A massive plexus consisting of pre- and postganglionic sympathetic, preganglionic parasympathetic, and visceral afferent fibers lies on the ventral surface of the abdominal aorta and continues onto its branches. Postganglionic sympathetic fibers (Fig. 13) from the celiac ganglia course through the celiac plexus which lies on the front and sides of the aorta at the levels of the origins of its celiac, superior mesenteric, and renal branches. Branches of this plexus extend along these arteries or their branches and are named accordingly: hepatic, gastric, splenic, suprarenal, etc. Postganglionic fibers from the superior mesenteric ganglion join the celiac plexus or continue along the superior mesenteric plexus. Through the celiac and superior mesenteric plexuses and their subsidiaries, all abdominal viscera except the descending colon receive postganglionic sympathetic fibers. (One exception is the suprarenal medulla which receives *preganglionic* sympathetic fibers via the celiac and suprarenal plexuses.)

The inferior mesenteric ganglion lies in its plexus at the origin of the inferior mesenteric artery and receives preganglionic fibers from the lumbar splanchnic nerves via the intermesenteric plexus. Postganglionic fibers enter the inferior mesenteric plexus and course to the descending colon along the branches of the inferior mesenteric artery. Other postganglionic fibers descend in front of the aorta as the superior hypogastric plexus (presacral nerve). This divides in front of the sacrum into the right and left hypogastric nerves or plexuses which continue inferiorly on each side of the rectum (and vagina in the female). At the lower part of the sacrum where the hypogastric nerves are joined by postganglionic nerves from the lower lumbar and sacral parts of the sympathetic trunks (via the lumbar and sacral splanchnic nerves), the hypogastric nerves become the inferior hypogastric (pelvic) plexus. Branches of the hypogastric plexuses accompany and are named after visceral branches of the internal iliac artery and supply the pelvic and perineal organs.

Parasympathetic Nerves

Parasympathetic preganglionic neurons are in the brain stem and spinal cord. These "craniosacral" neurons form visceral motor components in the oculomotor, facial, glossopharyngeal, and vagus nerve and in the middle three sacral spinal nerves (Fig. 14).

Oculomotor

The pupillary and lens responses associated with the light and accommodation reflexes are dependent upon parasympathetic fibers in the oculomotor nerves (Fig. 54).

Aggregates of small and medium-sized preganglionic-type neurons located in the periaqueductal gray on both sides of the median plane dorsomedial and rostral to the somatic oculomotor neurons, form the parasympathetic oculomotor nucleus of Edinger-Westphal.

The preganglionic fibers from these cells emerge in the interpeduncular fossa and pass to the orbit in the oculomotor nerves (Fig. 54). Within the orbit, the preganglionics enter the inferior division of the oculomotor nerve and its branch to the inferior oblique muscle. From here they form a single small branch or several tiny branches that enter the ciliary ganglion. These fibers synapse in this ganglion and are the only ones to do so.

Postganglionic fibers from the ciliary ganglion cells pass to the

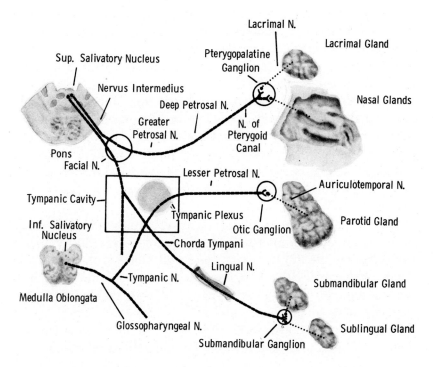

Figure 18. Illustration of VII and IX N. parasympathetics.

eye in the short ciliary nerves. After piercing the sclera, the fibers pass anteriorly along its inner surface and terminate on the ciliary and sphincter pupillae muscles.

Facial

Parasympathetic components of the facial nerve are secretomotor for the glands of the orbital, nasal, and oral cavities (Fig. 18).

Secretomotor cells scattered in the lateral reticular formation between the facial and vestibular nuclei form the superior salivatory nucleus. The preganglionic fibers from these neurons emerge in the nervus intermedius located in the cerebellopontine angle between the motor root of VII and the vestibulocochlear nerve. Within the facial canal, some of the preganglionic parasympathetic fibers form the greater petrosal nerve. This petrosal nerve passes toward the foramen lacerum, where it is joined by the deep petrosal nerve to form the nerve of the pterygoid canal which reaches the pterygopalatine ganglion. These preganglionic parasympathetic fibers form the only synapses in this ganglion.

Postganglionic parasympathetic fibers from the pterygopalatine ganglion accompany branches of the maxillary nerve to their destinations. The zygomatic and lacrimal branches carry them to the lacrimal gland, whereas the secretomotor fibers for the glands of the mucous membranes of the nasal cavity, palate, and pharynx travel with the nasal, palatine, and pharyngeal nerves.

The remaining preganglionic parasympathetic fibers of the facial nerve join the chorda tympani which leaves the tympanic cavity, enters the infratemporal fossa and unites with the lingual nerve. This carries them to their destination in the submandibular ganglion. These fibers synapse in this ganglion and are the only ones to do so.

Postganglionic fibers from the submandibular ganglion are then distributed to the submandibular and sublingual glands.

Glossopharyngeal

Parasympathetic components of the glossopharyngeal nerve are secretomotor for the parotid gland (Fig. 18). Preganglionic cells scattered medial to the nucleus solitarius in the rostral part of the medullary reticular formation form the inferior salivatory nucleus. The preganglionic fibers from these cells emerge in the glossopharyngeal nerve and enter its tympanic branch. Within the middle ear cavity these preganglionic fibers course through the tympanic plexus and reunite to form the lesser petrosal nerve. Upon emerging from the temporal bone into the middle cranial fossa, the lesser petrosal nerve passes to the infratemporal fossa through its own or an existing foramen and reaches the otic ganglion. These preganglionic parasympathetic fibers form the only synapses in this ganglion.

Postganglionic parasympathetic fibers emerge from the otic ganglion and pass via a communicating branch to the auriculotemporal nerve which distributes them to the parotid gland.

Vagus

Secreto- and visceromotor components of the vagus nerves are widely distributed and account for the parasympathetic influences on the thoracic viscera and all parasympathetically innervated abdominal viscera except the descending colon (Fig. 14).

Beneath the floor of the fourth ventricle and lateral to the hypoglossal nucleus is a conspicuous longitudinal aggregate of parasympathetic neurons, the dorsal nucleus of the vagus. Preganglionic fibers from these cells emerge from the brain stem in the postolivary sulcus. The vagus nerves leave the cranial cavity through the jugular foramen and descend within the carotid sheath to the thorax. After traveling through the superior mediastinum anterior to the subclavian artery on the right and the aortic arch on the left, the vagus nerves pass behind the root of the lung and onto the esophagus, and enter the abdomen. Cervical, thoracic, and abdominal branches carry preganglionic parasympathetic fibers to their synapses in terminal ganglia located in or near the target organs (Fig. 14).

Parasympathetic fibers in the cervical branches of the vagus are secretomotor for the pharynx, larynx, and trachea, and both secreto- and visceromotor for the esophagus. These preganglionic fibers, traveling in the pharyngeal, superior laryngeal, and recurrent laryngeal nerves synapse in ganglion cells in the pharyngeal plexus and in the extrinsic and/or intrinsic plexuses of the larynx, trachea, and esophagus. Postganglionic fibers from these terminal ganglia innervate the pharyngeal, laryngeal, and tracheal glands and the upper part of the esophagus.

Preganglionic parasympathetic fibers that influence the heart travel in the superior cervical cardiac branches from the cervical part, and the inferior cervical cardiac branches from the thoracic part of the vagus nerve. These fibers synapse on terminal ganglion cells located in the cardiac plexus and in the wall of the heart. Postganglionic parasympathetic fibers from these extrinsic and intrinsic cardiac ganglia innervate the auricles and conducting system.

Parasympathetic secreto- and visceromotor influences on the bronchi and lungs travel from the vagus nerves through their bronchial branches to the pulmonary plexuses. From here these preganglionic fibers enter the bronchi and bronchioles and synapse on ganglion cells located mainly in the deep plexuses within the walls of these structures. Postganglionic fibers from these intrinsic terminal ganglia innervate the smooth muscle and glands of the bronchial tree down to the respiratory bronchioles.

Below the root of the lung the vagus nerves enter the adventitial layer of the esophagus and join the esophageal plexus. Preganglionic parasympathetic fibers then pierce the wall of the esophagus and synapse on terminal ganglia in the myenteric plexus. Secreto- and visceromotor postganglionic parasympathetic fibers from these ganglion cells supply the glandular and muscular layers of the lower part of the esophagus.

Preganglionic parasympathetic fibers descend into the abdomen as the anterior and posterior vagal trunks which form from the esophageal plexus just above the diaphragm.

Preganglionic parasympathetic fibers destined for the abdominal viscera travel via the hepatic, gastric, and celiac branches of the vagal trunks. The hepatic branches join the hepatic plexuses through which parasympathetic secreto- and visceromotor fibers are distributed to terminal ganglia along or within the walls of the bile ducts and gall bladder. The gastric branches fan out from the cardia and spread over the fundus and body of the stomach. Along their route these preganglionic parasympathetic fibers penetrate the stomach wall and are distributed to terminal ganglia in the myenteric and submucous plexuses. Viscero- and secretomotor postganglionic fibers from these ganglion cells terminate in the muscular coats and gastric glands.

Parasympathetic fibers remaining in the vagal trunks distal to their gastric and hepatic branches, join the celiac plexus. These viscero- and secretomotor preganglionic fibers pass *without synapsing* through the celiac and its subsidiary plexuses to the pancreas and to the gastrointestinal tract as far caudad as the splenic flexure. Terminal ganglia within the pancreatic interlobular septa and within the myenteric and submucous plexuses of the stomach and intestines send postganglionic parasympathetic fibers to the glands and muscular coats of these organs.

Sacral

Parasympathetic influences on defecation, micturition, and erection are mediated through sacral and pelvic nerves to extrinsic or intrinsic terminal ganglia associated with the appropriate organs (Fig. 14).

Groups of small and medium-sized preganglionic-type neurons located dorsally in the spinal intermediate gray next to the lateral funiculus form an intermediolateral column of cells usually extending from the caudal part of S.2 to the rostral part of S.4. Preganglionic fibers from these cells emerge from the spinal cord mainly in the ventral roots of S.3 and 4 and occasionally in those of S.2 or 5.

These parasympathetic fibers travel in the ventral rami and upon entering the pelvic cavity through the sacral foramina, form the pelvic splanchnic nerves (nervi erigentes) which join the inferior hypogastric (pelvic) plexuses.

Preganglionic parasympathetic fibers destined for the distal parts of the colon and the rectum pass through plexuses or individual retroperitoneal nerves that arise from the inferior and superior hypogastric plexuses and carry them to the descending and sigmoid parts of the colon and the superior part of the rectum. The middle rectal plexus from the inferior hypogastric plexus supplies the lower part of the rectum and the anal canal. Upon reaching their target organs, these preganglionic fibers penetrate the walls and synapse on ganglion cells in the myenteric and submucous plexuses. Postganglionic secreto- and visceromotor fibers from these myenteric and submucous ganglia then terminate on the glands and the smooth muscle of the descending colon, sigmoid colon, rectum, and anal canal.

Parasympathetic fibers that influence the ureter and bladder pass from the inferior hypogastric plexus to the vesical plexus. These preganglionic fibers synapse on ganglia either in the vesical plexus or in the walls of the bladder and lower third of the ureters. Postganglionic fibers from these terminal ganglion cells innervate the smooth muscle of the ureter and bladder. Parasympathetic influences on the erectile tissue of the penis and vagina and the glands of the genital system travel via preganglionic fibers in the inferior hypogastric plexus to terminal ganglia located within this plexus and within the prostatic plexus in the male and the vesical plexus in the female. Postganglionic fibers from the prostatic plexus innervate the bulbourethral glands and then follow the urethra through the pelvic diaphragm as cavernous nerves to the helicine arteries in the corpora cavernosa of the penis. Postganglionic fibers from the uterovaginal plexus follow the female urethra as cavernous nerves to the erectile tissue of the clitoris and of the vestibule.

Functional Characteristics of the Autonomic System

Most of the visceral organs have a dual nerve supply, one from the sympathetic and one from the parasympathetic system (Fig. 19). During their peripheral course, the nerve fibers of the parasympathetic and sympathetic systems are intermingled, but they retain their functional independence. Some tissues are innervated by only one division. The peripheral blood vessels, the pilomotor muscles, the spleen, and the sweat glands receive a single innervation from the sympathetic division. Table V summarizes the actions of autonomic nerves on various organs.

The sympathetic and parasympathetic systems integrate and are complementary. Both of them take part in the intricate regulation of visceral functions, ensuring proper adjustment for normal functioning. This influence is not limited to adjusting them only in respect to each other, since adjustments to somatic functions also occur. The entire sympathetic system goes into action as a unit throughout the body for sustained periods of time. Under stress situations, the suprarenal medulla is also stimulated to release epinephrine into the bloodstream for diffuse distribution. This facilitates the mass action of the sympathetic division.

Cannon said that sympathetic nerves prepare the body for "fight or flight" in emergency situations. To meet the situation, the sympathetic system acts to supply more blood to the skeletal muscles, rich in oxygen and glucose. The heart rate increases and the blood vessels constrict, in particular those blood vessels leading to the skin and the viscera, thereby shunting the

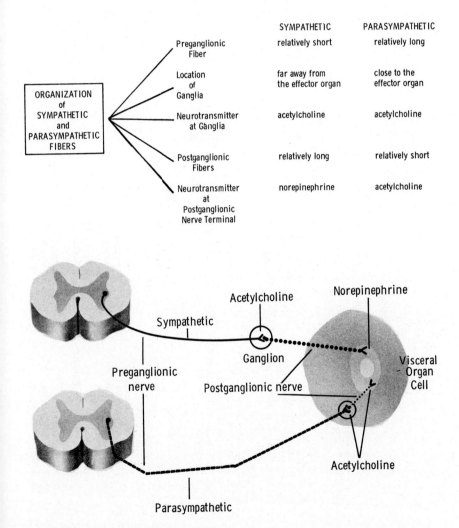

Figure 19. Organization of sympathetic and parasympathetic fibers.

TABLE V

COMPARISON OF SYMPATHETIC AND PARASYMPATHETIC SYSTEMS

Structure or function	Sympathetic	Parasympathetic
I. Anatomical		
A. Outflow from CNS	Thoracolumbar	Craniosacral
B. Location of ganglia	Closer to CNS	Closer to effector organs
C. Pre- to post-ggl**** neurons	More post-ggl	Ratio closer to 1
D. Distribution of effectors	Throughout the body	More limited
II. Functional		
A. Cardiac muscle		
1. Heart rate	Increases	Decreases
2. Force of ventr. contr.	Increases	No direct effect
3. A–V node and conduction system	Increases conduction velocity	Decreases conduction velocity, A–V block
B. Smooth muscle		
1. Blood vessels	Constriction usually*	Little effect**
2. Iris	Pupillary dilatation	Pupillary constriction
3. Bronchi	Dilatation	Constriction
4. Gastrointestinal tract		
a. Motility and tone	Decreases	Increases
b. Sphincters	Contraction	Relaxation
5. Gallbladder and ducts	Relaxation	Contraction
6. Urinary bladder		
a. Detrusor	Relaxation (?)	Contraction
b. Trigone and sphincter	Contraction	Relaxation
7. Uterus	Variable	Variable
8. Sex organs	Ejaculation	Erection
9. Pilomotor muscles	Contraction	—
10. Spleen capsule	Contraction	—

C. Glands
  1. Salivary glands — Secretion (scanty, viscous) — Secretion (watery)
  2. Gastrointestinal glands — Inhibition*** — Secretion
  3. Sweat glands — Secretion* — —
  4. Suprarenal medulla — Secretion* —

D. Metabolism
  1. Liver — Glycogenolysis — —
  2. Adipose tissue — Free fatty acid release — —

E. General homeostasis — Combat or emergency, energy mobilization — Protection, conservation and restoration of resources

III. Chemical
  A. Neuroeffector transmitter — Mostly norepinephrine* — Acetylcholine
  B. Destruction of transmitter — Slow — Rapid
  C. Synthesis of transmitter — Slow — Rapid
  D. Systemic reinforcement — Secretion of norepinephrine and epinephrine by suprarenal medulla — —

---

* Sympathetic neuroeffector transmission is mediated by acetylcholine in some blood vessels of skeletal muscle, in the sweat glands, and in the suprarenal medulla.
** Some blood vessels in the facial and pelvic regions are dilated by parasympathetic impulses.
*** In most cases.
**** Ganglion.

blood into the dilated vessels of the skeletal muscles. The bronchioles dilate to facilitate the entry of more air. The pupil of the eye dilates and the body hair "stands on end." The gastrointestinal tract relaxes and digestion is postponed until the emergency is over. The gastrointestinal sphincters contract to prevent continued digestion. Glycogen is broken down into glucose and blood sugar rises. Thus the sympathetic system is concerned with the mobilization of energy during emergency and stress situations. The sympathetic division is not vital for life under normal conditions, but it is critical for the proper reaction to stress and strain.

Unlike the widespread actions of the sympathetic system, the parasympathetic system is more localized in its actions. Typically, it affects a single organ or in some cases small groups of organs, without affecting others. The response is relatively of short duration. The main functions of the parasympathetic nerves are conservation and restoration of the energy stores of the body and excretion of waste products. The cranial portion is known as the "conserver of bodily resources" and the sacral portion as the "mechanism of emptying." It is active during the calm, steady, and homeostatic state.

Cannon said: "The sympathetics are like the loud and soft pedals, modulating all the notes together; the cranial and sacral innervations are like the separate keys."

The sympathetic and parasympathetic systems are continually active, and the basal rate of activity is known respectively as sympathetic tone and parasympathetic tone. For example, sympathetic tone normally keeps almost all the blood vessels of the body constricted to approximately one-half their maximum diameter. By increasing tone, the vessels can be constricted even more. On the other hand, by inhibiting the normal tone, the vessels can be dilated. Another example of tone is that exerted by the parasympathetic system in the gastrointestinal tract. Surgical removal of parasympathetic innervation, e.g. vagotomy, can cause serious and prolonged "atony."

CHAPTER 3

VISCERAL INPUT AND
CENTRAL AUTONOMIC COMPONENTS

Visceral Afferent Nerves

PERIPHERAL NERVES CARRYING autonomic pre- and postganglionic fibers to the viscera and blood vessels, also contain nerve fibers carrying visceral impulses in the opposite direction, i.e. toward the brain and spinal cord. These are the general visceral afferent fibers or the autonomic afferent fibers responsible for visceral input. Such afferent fibers are the myelinated and unmyelinated peripheral branches coming from axons of unipolar neurons located in spinal and cranial nerve ganglia. Although these fibers are distributed mainly with the parasympathetic and sympathetic nerves and plexuses, they *never synapse* in the autonomic ganglia.

The importance of impulses arising from visceral organs and blood vessels is mainly the initiation of visceral reflexes; most do not reach the level of consciousness. Those autonomic afferent impulses that do reach levels of awareness result in sensations that are vague and poorly localized, e.g. hunger, nausea, distension of urinary bladder and rectum, sexual sensations. In certain conditions visceral sensations become painful and are medically important.

Visceral organs including the brain and spinal cord are in-

51

sensitive to ordinary mechanical and thermal stimuli. Thus, even though handling, cutting, crushing, or burning of viscera occurs during surgical procedures, sensations are not elicited. Painful sensations do result from excessive stretch, violent or spastic contractions, or decreased blood supply. In such conditions the pain may be felt in the region of the organ itself (true visceral pain), or in a region of skin or other somatic tissue innervated by the same spinal cord or brain stem level that receives the visceral afferent impulses (referred pain).

Various forms of free and encapsulated nerve endings in viscera and in the walls of blood vessels are the receptors for visceral input. Such input occurs mainly via certain cranial and spinal nerves. The glossopharyngeal, vagus, and second, third, and fourth sacral nerves distribute visceral afferent fibers along parasympathetic paths, whereas the thoracic and upper lumbar spinal nerves distribute them through communicating rami to sympathetic nerves and peripheral blood vessels. In general, those fibers associated with reflex control of visceral activity accompany the parasympathetic nerves, whereas those that convey visceral sensations accompany the sympathetic nerves. An exception to this are visceral pain fibers from certain pelvic viscera (sigmoid colon, rectum, neck of bladder, prostate gland, and cervix of uterus) that accompany the pelvic parasympathetic nerves.

Cranial Pathways

The glossopharyngeal nerve carries visceral afferent impulses arising mainly from the mucous membrane of the posterior part of the tongue, the tonsil and pharynx, and from the carotid sinus and body. Impulses from these play a major role in reflexes associated with deglutition, gaging, circulation, and respiration. The cell bodies are in the ganglia of the glossopharyngeal nerve and central connections are made through the tractus solitarius.

The vagus nerve distributes visceral afferent fibers to all parts of the digestive tube from the pharynx to as far distal as the splenic flexure, to the heart and the walls of the great vessels and aortic bodies, and to the walls of the bronchial tree and interalveolar tissue of the lungs. The vagal visceral afferent fibers initiate gastrointestinal, cardiovascular, and respiratory reflexes. Their cell bodies are in the inferior (nodose) ganglion and central connections are made through the tractus solitarius and its nucleus.

The tractus solitarius extends from the lower part of the pons to the obex and is closely related throughout its course to the solitary nucleus. The primary fibers in the solitary tract synapse in the solitary nucleus; secondary fibers enter the reticular formation through which connections are made with the respiratory and cardiovascular centers, visceral and somatic motor nuclei, and higher centers.

Spinal Pathways (*Table VI*)

Visceral afferent impulses course in the sacral parasympathetic nerves from the pelvic viscera. Receptors in the sigmoid colon, rectum, urinary bladder, proximal part of the urethra, and cervix of the uterus transform stimuli into visceral afferent impulses subserving reflexes and sensations. Some of these fibers course in the pelvic splanchnic nerves and have their cell bodies located in the dorsal root ganglia of the second, third, and fourth sacral spinal nerves. Others travel through the inferior hypogastric plexus, hypogastric nerves, superior hypogastric plexus, lumbar splanchnic nerves, and sympathetic trunk to reach their cells of origin in the dorsal root ganglia of the lower thoracic and upper lumbar spinal nerves.

A similar double innervation occurs in the thoracic and abdominal viscera: a parasympathetic path funneled through the vagus nerves and a sympathetic funneled through the sympathetic trunks. From the heart, coronary vessels, bronchial tree and lungs, visceral afferent fibers travel in the cardiac and pulmonary nerves to the sympathetic trunk. From the abdominal viscera, afferent fibers travel through the mesenteric and celiac plexuses, and the thoracic and lumbar splanchnic nerves to the sympathetic trunk. After an uninterrupted course these afferent fibers enter the thoracic and upper lumbar spinal nerves through the white communicating rami and reach their cell bodies located in the dorsal root ganglia of T.1 through L.2.

VISCERAL PAIN PATHS

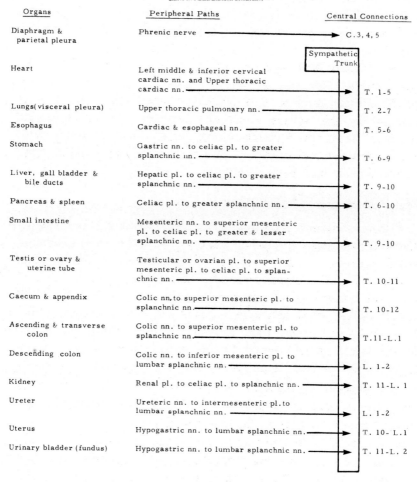

Organs	Peripheral Paths	Central Connections
Diaphragm & parietal pleura	Phrenic nerve	C. 3, 4, 5
Heart	Left middle & inferior cervical cardiac nn. and Upper thoracic cardiac nn.	T. 1-5
Lungs(visceral pleura)	Upper thoracic pulmonary nn.	T. 2-7
Esophagus	Cardiac & esophageal nn.	T. 5-6
Stomach	Gastric nn. to celiac pl. to greater splanchnic nn.	T. 6-9
Liver, gall bladder & bile ducts	Hepatic pl. to celiac pl. to greater splanchnic nn.	T. 9-10
Pancreas & spleen	Celiac pl. to greater splanchnic nn.	T. 6-10
Small intestine	Mesenteric nn. to superior mesenteric pl. to celiac pl. to greater & lesser splanchnic nn.	T. 9-10
Testis or ovary & uterine tube	Testicular or ovarian pl. to superior mesenteric pl. to celiac pl. to splanchnic nn.	T. 10-11
Caecum & appendix	Colic nn. to superior mesenteric pl. to splanchnic nn.	T. 10-12
Ascending & transverse colon	Colic nn. to superior mesenteric pl. to splanchnic nn.	T. 11-L. 1
Descending colon	Colic nn. to inferior mesenteric pl. to lumbar splanchnic nn.	L. 1-2
Kidney	Renal pl. to celiac pl. to splanchnic nn.	T. 11-L. 1
Ureter	Ureteric nn. to intermesenteric pl. to lumbar splanchnic nn.	L. 1-2
Uterus	Hypogastric nn. to lumbar splanchnic nn.	T. 10- L.1
Urinary bladder (fundus)	Hypogastric nn. to lumbar splanchnic nn.	T. 11-L. 2

Sympathetic Trunk

| Urinary bladder (neck), Urethra, prostate gland, cervix of uterus, sigmoid colon, and rectum | Pelvic splanchnic nn. | S. 2-4 |

The phrenic nerve also contains visceral afferent fibers coming from the pericardium, diaphragm, hepatic ligaments and capsule, pancreas, and suprarenal glands. Visceral afferent fibers from peripheral blood vessels probably travel centrally in all spinal nerves. In both cases the cell bodies of these autonomic afferent components are unipolar neurons in appropriate dorsal root ganglia.

Regardless of their route from the thoracic, abdominal, or pelvic cavities, or from blood vessels, visceral afferent fibers make their first synapse in the spinal cord. The fibers enter the cord through the lateral division of the dorsal root and synapse on cells located in the posterior horn and intermediate zone. Those impulses associated with the initiation of visceral or somatic reflexes make secondary connections with visceral or somatic motor neurons in the lateral or anterior horns of the spinal gray matter (Figs. 11–12). Those visceral impulses destined to reach conscious levels, ascend bilaterally in the anterolateral quadrants and upon reaching the brain stem, continue through multisynaptic pathways in the reticular formation to higher centers.

Visceral Sensation and Referred Pain

Although viscera are relatively insensitive, exaggerated stretching or contraction of smooth muscle and certain pathological conditions will elicit awareness, discomfort, or pain. True visceral sensations, e.g. heartburn, nausea, hunger, fullness of bladder and rectum, sexual sensations, tend to be vague and poorly localized. This is probably due to such characteristics as their multisynaptic central pathways and the meager representation of viscera in the sensory areas of the cerebral cortex.

More often in pathological conditions visceral pain has a tendency to irradiate to cutaneous areas, and therefore, is assumed by the patient to arise mainly or exclusively in surface areas of the body; hence the term "referred pain." It is important to recall that most visceral pain fibers travel with sympathetic nerves and reach the thoracic and upper lumbar spinal nerves through the fourteen pairs of white rami communicating with the sympathetic trunks. Thus, while the region to which the pain is referred may, at first sight, seem unrelated to the pathological visceral organ, the two loci are part of the same segmental level.

The commonly accepted explanation for referred pain is that within the spinal gray matter, the visceral afferent impulses converge on secondary somatic afferent neurons and lower their threshold. Thus, an abnormally large volley of visceral afferent impulses causes somatic afferent neurons to fire, resulting in deception of the cerebral cortex.

Central Autonomic Components

Although sympathetic and parasympathetic preganglionic neurons are limited to nuclei localized at thoracolumbar and craniosacral levels, they may be influenced by neurons at other levels. Thus, many types of autonomic phenomena have been associated with various parts of the cerebral hemispheres, e.g. frontal lobe, cingulate gyrus, orbital-insular-temporal cortex, hippocampus, amygdala, caudate nucleus. Most of the visceral responses are diffuse and tend to overlap somatic reactions. Also, all seem to be mediated through the hypothalamus.

Hypothalamus

Although visceral activity may be elicited by stimulation of neuronal centers located in the brain stem, cerebellum, and cerebral cortex, the highest center for the integration of autonomic activity is the hypothalamus. Multisynaptic paths from this part of the diencephalon descend through the brain stem reticular formation and the spinal cord reticulospinal tracts to regulate body temperature, blood pressure, digestion, respiration, etc. In addition to its integration of autonomic functions, the hypothalamus also influences water balance, the endocrine glands, the sleep-waking cycle, and emotions.

STRUCTURE. The hypothalamus is the most ventral part of the diencephalon and can be observed on the base of the brain.

Medially it forms the walls of the lower part of the third ventricle and extends dorsally as far as the hypothalamic sulcus which separates hypothalamus from thalamus. Anteriorly it extends to the lamina terminalis where it blends with the preoptic area. Laterally it blends with the subthalamus and posteriorly it is continuous with the midbrain tegmentum.

For descriptive purposes the hypothalamus is divided into three parts, anterior, intermediate, and posterior. The anterior part is at the level of the optic chiasm and is called the supraoptic region. The intermediate part is at the level of the tuber cinereum and infundibulum, and is called the tuberal region. The posterior part is at the mamillary bodies and is called the mamillary region. In addition to this antero-posterior division, the hypothalamus is frequently divided into periventricular, medial and lateral parts. The latter two are separated by the fornix.

INPUT (Fig. 20A). All parts of the central nervous system influence hypothalamic activity. In addition, non-neural stimuli, e.g. alterations in osmotic pressure and temperature of blood, can stimulate hypothalamic neurons directly.

Ascending impulses such as pain and taste, reach the hypothalamus from the brain stem reticular formation by way of the mamillary peduncle which projects to the posterior part of the hypothalamus. Secondary olfactory connections from the septal region enter the hypothalamus in the medial forebrain bundle. Through these connections sensory input may elicit autonomic activities associated with salivation, nausea, appetite, etc.

From the amygdaloid nucleus impulses may reach the hypothalamus, either through the stria terminalis which passes in the groove next to the caudate nucleus and enters the anterior hypothalamus, or through the ansa peduncularis which emerges from the inferior amygdala, loops under the lenticular nucleus and internal capsule and invades the hypothalamus from its ventrolateral aspect.

The hippocampal formation influences the hypothalamus, chiefly the more posterior parts, by way of the fornix. Through this connection it is thought that memory and alertness are influenced by posterior hypothalamic activity.

The prefrontal cortex influences the hypothalamus either directly by fibers passing from posterior orbital regions to the

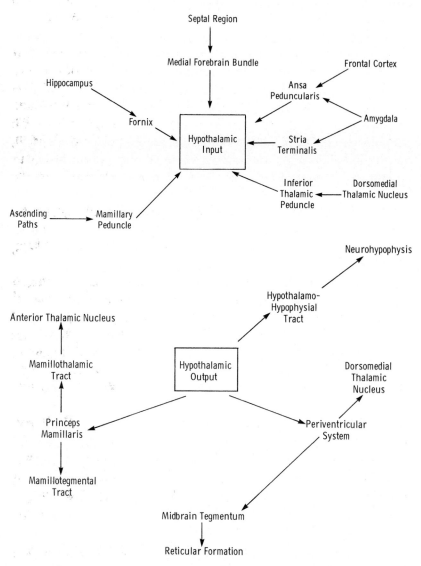

Figure 20 A and B. Connections of the hypothalamus.

anterior hypothalamus via the ansa peduncularis, or from lateral prefrontal regions by synapsing in the dorsomedial nucleus of the thalamus which then connects to the hypothalamus through the inferior thalamic peduncle. It is thought that the hypothalamus expresses the emotions that are perceived in these cortical areas.

OUTPUT (Fig. 20B). Unlike input, there is a fairly limited distribution of efferent projections from the hypothalamus.

From the mamillary region arises a very distinct bundle, the princeps mamillaris which passes dorsally and divides into tegmental and thalamic tracts. The mamillotegmental tract enters the tegmentum and influences the midbrain reticular formation. This provides a "meeting place" where hypothalamic activity can contact the ascending reticular activating system, both of which are thought to play important roles in the activation of the cerebral cortex. The mamillothalamic tract projects to the anterior nucleus of the thalamus. This is part of the Papez circuit that is thought to influence neocortical

Region	Nucleus	Function	Lesion
Anterior or Supraoptic	1. Supraoptic	Water Conservation ADH Production and Release	Diabetes Insipidus Diuresis
	2. Paraventricular	" Thirst Center Oxytocin Release	" Abnormal Water Intake Oxytocin Decrease
	3. Preoptic	Thermal Sensitivity Parasympathomimetic	Hyperthermia
Intermediate or Tuberal	1. Dorsomedial	Gastrointestinal Muscular and Glandular Activity	Decreased GI Activity
	2. Ventromedial	Behavior	Rage Reaction
	3. Lateral	" Food Intake	" Anorexia
Posterior or Mamillary	Posterior	Body Temperature Sympathomimetic	Poikilothermia
	Mamillary	Cortical Activity	Unknown

Figure 21. Functions of hypothalamic nuclei

activity and to have a very strong relationship to the storage of recent memory.

A periventricular system of fibers passes along the wall of the third ventricle and is distributed to the dorsomedial nucleus of the thalamus and the periaqueductal gray of the midbrain. Such connections with the dorsomedial nucleus of the thalamus allow strong influences with the prefrontal cortex. The periaqueductal gray connections become incorporated into the dorsal longitudinal fasciculus and the reticular formation of the midbrain. These descending impulses allow the hypothalamus to influence the various visceral and somatic centers in the brain stem and spinal cord.

A third group of fibers consists of the hypothalamo-hypophyseal tracts. These unmyelinated fibers arise chiefly from the supraoptic and paraventricular nuclei and provide a pathway for the axonal migration of antidiuretic hormone which is formed within these neurons and transported to the neural hypophysis by their axons.

A vascular channel also plays an important role in hypothalamic output. This consists of the hypophyseal portal system. The anterior lobe of the pituitary receives its blood supply from this system. Hypophyseal branches of the internal carotid arteries form a ring around the infundibulum. Branches from this ring invade the stalk of the pituitary as sinusoidal capillaries. Through this vascular connection hypothalamic neurons influence the activity of the endocrine glands. It is thought that the hypothalamus produces activating agents or releasing factors which are absorbed into the hypophyseal portal system and transported to the secretory cells within the adenohypophysis. The functions of the hypothalamic nuclei are summarized in Figure 21.

Descending Pathways

Pathways from the hypothalamus to autonomic centers and neurons in the brain stem and spinal cord are not clearly known. In the midbrain and rostral pons such descending paths seem to be located dorsomedially, i.e. near the periaqueductal gray and floor of the fourth ventricle. Some evidence exists that from these areas the paths sweep laterally and descend through the caudal pons and the medulla in the lateral part of the reticular formation. Various degrees of Horner's syndrome may occur with unilateral lesions in the dorsolateral part of the medulla.

The spinal course of descending autonomic impulses involves reticulospinal fibers in the anterolateral quadrant and perhaps the anterior funiculus.

Autonomic Centers

In addition to the hypothalamic nuclei, other groups of neurons at various levels strongly influence autonomic activities. At the level of the midbrain, centers for pupillary responses are located in the pretectal area and superior colliculus. In the pons, a pneumotaxic center near the locus ceruleus and an apneustic center in the reticular formation at more caudal levels influence respiration. In the medulla are the vital vasomotor and respiratory centers.

Although these various centers receive input from many sources, (hypothalamus, cranial nerves, ascending pathways, etc.) their output is funneled to autonomic and, in some cases, associated somatic neurons. For details on the locations and connections of some of the more important centers, see Table VII.

TABLE VII

IMPORTANT CENTERS AND THEIR CONNECTIONS

FUNCTION	LOCATION	CENTRAL PATHS	EFFERENT PATHS
Vasomotor Pressor	Lat. Reticular Formation deep to Inferior Fovea	Reticulospinal	Intermediolateral Nucleus to Sympathetic Ganglia
Depressor	Med. Reticular Formation at Obex	Reticulovagal	Dorsal Vagal Nucleus to Cardiac Ganglia
Respiratory* Inspiratory	Ventromedial Reticular Formation at Inf. Olivary Nucl.	Reticulospinal	*Motoneurons C. 3, 4, 5 to Diaphragm
Expiratory	Dorsolateral Reticular Formation at Inf. Olivary Nucl.	Reticuloreticular	
Vomiting	Reticular Formation at Obex	Reticulovagal	Dorsal Vagal Nucleus to Gastric Enteric Ganglia
		Reticulospinal	Intermediolateral Nucleus T. 6–10 to Pylorus via Celiac Ganglion
		Reticulospinal	*Motoneurons to Diaphragm & Abdominal Muscles
Micturition	Frontal lobe (?) Hypothalamus (?)	Corticospinal (?) Reticulospinal (?)	1) *Motoneurons S. 2, 3, 4 to Pelvic Diaphragm or Urethral Sphincter 2) Intermediolateral Nucleus S. 2, 3, 4 to Detrusor via Vesical Ganglia
Defecation	Frontal lobe (?) Hypothalamus (?)	Corticospinal (?) Reticulospinal (?)	1) *Motoneurons S. 2, 3, 4 to Anal Sphincter 2) Intermediolateral Nucleus S. 2, 3, 4 to Enteric Ganglia of Colon and Rectum

* Not Autonomic

CHAPTER 4

CHEMICAL TRANSMISSION

Development of Transmitter Concept

THERE IS A SIMILARITY between the effects of drugs and those of nerve stimulation. For example, when muscarine is applied to the heart, it slows it in a manner similar to vagal stimulation. In 1895, Oliver and Schaffer showed that the adrenal medullary extract mimicked the effects of sympathetic stimulation. Therefore, they suggested that sympathetic nerves may act by releasing a chemical substance. Although this idea was interesting, it was not universally accepted. Elliot, in 1905, wrote: "The reaction to adrenaline on any plain muscle in the body is of a similar character to that following excitation of the sympathetic nerves supplying that muscle," and further, that "when plain muscle develops connections with sympathetic nerves, it must at the myoneural junction acquire a mechanism that can receive the nervous impulse and thereupon initiate the appropriate muscular response. That part of the junction which is irritated by adrenaline is on the muscular side."

However, the convincing evidence that chemical transmission occurs was provided by Loewi in 1921. He perfused two isolated frog hearts with Ringer's solution in such a way that the solution flowed through one heart and then perfused the other. When the vagus nerve of the first heart was stimulated, the

63

heart slowed and shortly afterward, the second heart behaved in a similar manner. On the basis of these results, he suggested that during stimulation of the vagus, a substance which slowed the first heart was released from the nerve endings. When this substance was carried in perfusion fluid to the second heart, it arrested the second heart also. He called this substance "vagus-stoff." He pointed out that this substance is released in a minute quantity, is extremely potent and is hydrolyzed by a specific enzyme, cholinesterase. By similar experiments he was also able to show that stimulation of the "nervus accelerans" (cardiac sympathetics) caused the release of an accelerator substance called "acceleranstoff." Subsequent work established the fact that the "vagustoff" was acetylcholine and "acceleranstoff" was epinephrine. Von Euler, in 1946, produced convincing evidence that in mammals the normal adrenergic transmitter at the post-ganglionic sympathetic nerve endings is norepinephrine, not epinephrine. Significant amounts of epinephrine also come from the suprarenals. The suprarenal gland produces both norepinephrine and epinephrine. The neurotransmission in the autonomic system and at the neuromuscular junction is essentially the same.

Criteria for Chemical Transmitters

On the basis of classical studies in the peripheral nervous system the following criteria are necessary for a substance to be classified as a chemical transmitter:

1. The substance and the enzyme system for its synthesis must be present at presynaptic sites.
2. The substance must be released from the presynaptic site in response to and in proportion to depolarization of the presynaptic membrane.
3. There must be a system for the inactivation of the released candidate transmitter. This could include an enzyme system for the destruction of the released candidate transmitter, or also a specific uptake mechanism for the reabsorption of the transmitter into the pre- or postsynaptic sites.

4. The substance must activate the postsynaptic sites, and it should mimic the actions of the neurally-released transmitter.

5. Agents which modify the actions of the neurally-released transmitter must affect the action of the substance in an identical manner.

Sequence of Chemical Events in Junctional Transmission

In junctional transmission, the sequence of chemical events is as follows:

1. *Synthesis and storage of the neurotransmitter.* Neurotransmitters are synthesized from precursors within the neurons and are stored in bound form in synaptic vesicles.

2. *Release of the transmitter.* Under resting conditions, there is a spontaneous random discharge of packets or quanta of the transmitter which sets up junctional potentials in the effector cells. The amount released is far too small to cause initiation of propagated impulses at the postsynaptic site. Arrival of an impulse causes depolarization and triggers the synchronous release of several quanta. It is believed that entry of a calcium ion may activate the discharge of the contents of the vesicles.

3. *Interaction with receptors.* The transmitter diffuses through the synaptic cleft and combines with receptive sites or receptors in the postjunctional membrane and causes an increase in the ionic permeability of the membrane, resulting in localized depolarization.

4. *Initiation of postsynaptic activity.* When the localized action potential reaches a critical level, it initiates a propagated action potential in the smooth muscle, resulting in a mechanical response.

5. *Inactivation of the transmitter.* The neurotransmitter is inactivated by a specific enzyme and may diffuse away from the site of its action or may be taken up again by the nerve.

6. *Repolarization of the postsynaptic membrane.* Inactivation of the neurotransmitter allows the repolarization of the postsynaptic membrane.

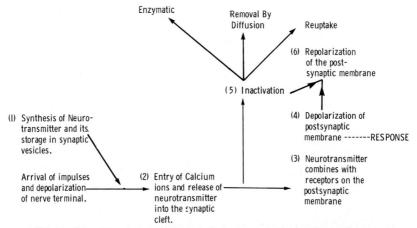

Figure 22a. Sequence of chemical events in junctional transmission

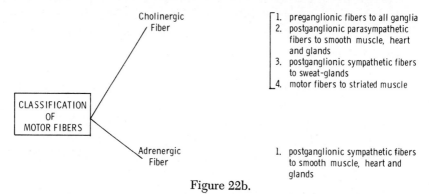

Figure 22b.

The main events in chemical transmission are summarized in Figure 22.

Neurotransmission in Suprarenal Medulla and Sweat Glands

The suprarenal medulla is derived embryologically from the same neural crest tissue as are autonomic ganglia. Therefore, the suprarenal gland is considered as a sympathetic ganglion which has lost its postganglionic sympathetic axons. It is innervated by splanchnic nerves which are preganglionic. On stimulation of the splanchnic nerves, the suprarenal medulla releases epinephrine. In order to study the mechanism of release of epinephrine, Feldberg and Minz in 1933 cannulated the lumbar vein of the left suprarenal gland of an anesthetized dog. The lumbar vein passes over the suprarenal gland and carries the blood leaving the suprarenal gland to the inferior vena cava. To prevent the destruction of any acetylcholine released in response to splanchnic nerve stimulation, these investigators injected eserine into the animal. They collected the blood before and during nerve stimulation. They found that samples collected before splanchnic nerve stimulation did not contain acetylcholine, whereas the samples collected during splanchnic nerve stimulation contain acetylcholine. On the basis of these

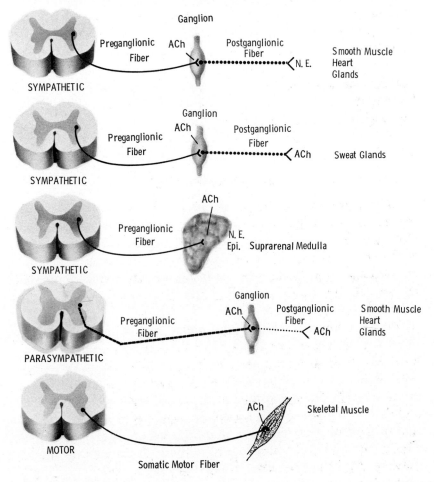

findings, they concluded that the splanchnic nerves innervating the suprarenal medulla released acetylcholine which in turn liberated epinephrine.

Sweat glands receive sympathetic innervation. Atropine inhibits sweating. Atropine blocks only the parasympathetic effects and not the sympathetic effects. Dale and Feldberg found that when the sympathetic fibers to sweat glands were stimulated, acetylcholine was released. The response was potentiated by eserine which prolongs the actions of acetylcholine by preventing its destruction by cholinesterase, and the response was abolished after atropine administration. Thus, they concluded that sympathetic fibers to sweat glands release acetylcholine rather than an epinephrine-like substance.

Dale called the nerve fibers that release acetylcholine, "cholinergic" and those that release epinephrine-like substances "adrenergic." Thus, postganglionic sympathetic fibers to the sweat glands and preganglionic fibers innervating the suprarenal glands are both cholinergic (Fig. 23A,B).

False Neurotransmitter

The processes for synthesis, storage, and release of neurotransmitter are not entirely specific. Structurally related compounds also may be formed which are stored in the synaptic vesicles and may be released by nerve stimulation. They act as a false neurotransmitter. If the false transmitter has reduced physiological activity, there may be a failure of transmission at the neuroeffector junction.

Triethylcholine is structurally similar to choline. In choline three methyl groups are attached to the nitrogen atom, whereas in triethylcholine the nitrogen has three ethyl groups. When triethylcholine is administered, choline acetylase makes the acetic ester of triethylcholine instead of the acetic ester of choline. The acetylated compound is released in response to nerve stimulation instead of acetylcholine. Since the acetic ester of triethylcholine has reduced physiological activity, it impairs the transmission. For example, when triethylcholine is added to a bath containing a phrenic nerve-diaphragm preparation, the response to nerve stimulation is reduced. On addition of choline, the response to nerve stimulation is restored.

Out of three enzymes responsible for formation of norepinephrine from tyrosine, only the first enzyme, tyrosine hydroxylase, is relatively specific. The other two enzymes, dopa-decarboxylase and dopamine-β-oxidase, are relatively non-specific.

Several amino acids such as α-methyl dopa and α-methyl-m-tyrosine can be taken up by adrenergic nerve endings following their administration, decarboxylated by dopa-decarboxylase, and subsequently taken up by granular vesicles where they are β-hydroxylated by dopamine-β-oxidase. These β-hydroxylated compounds act as false neurotransmitters (Fig. 24). They are released by nerve stimulation as well as by drugs which deplete norepinephrine.

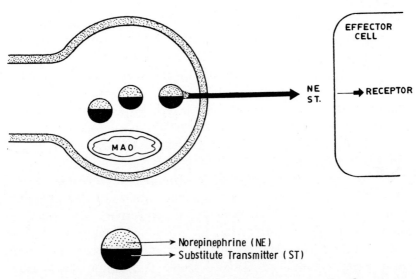

Figure 24. *Diagrammatic illustration of transmitter released in the presence of a substitute transmitter.* Foreign amine derived from α-Methyl Dopa and α-Methyl-M-Tyrosine may replace Norepinephrine in the storage vesicles and act as a false transmitter. Replacement of Norepinephrine by a substitute transmitter results in a diminished release of Norepinephrine and therefore apparent adrenergic blockade.

CHAPTER 5

AUTONOMIC NERVE TERMINALS

A^{S A POSTGANGLIONIC AXON} approaches the smooth muscle it innervates, it is distributed in a network of terminations which lack the specificity of the neuromuscular junction seen in the motor end-plate of somatic axons and skeletal muscle. The autonomic axons have two main characteristics:

1. The ramification of terminals are longer than the smooth muscles being innervated.
2. In most cases, especially in the sympathetic system, there is multiple innervation or overlap so that a smooth muscle cell may be innervated from terminals of a number of different axons.

Recently it has been possible to examine the anatomic distribution of sympathetic postganglionic fibers in considerable detail. With the development of sensitive histochemical methods, specific identification of adrenergic neurons has become possible. The sympathetic postganglionic fibers arise from nerve cells in the sympathetic trunk and autonomic plexus ganglia. From each cell body a "long" unmyelinated axon arises. It is usually 0.2 to 1 μ in diameter. These "long" axons provide innervation to smooth muscle and glands in many organs. There is also a system of adrenergic neurons whose cell bodies are located more peripherally, that is, in ganglia close to or within the pelvic organs. From the nerve cells in these ganglia arise "short" adrenergic axons that innervate the accessory male genital organs, parts of the female reproductive tract, the urethra, and the trigonal area of the urinary bladder (Fig. 25).

When the postganglionic axon approaches the tissue to be innervated, it becomes varicose. In the innervated tissue each axon splits into a system of branches called nerve terminals (Fig. 26). The terminal fibers of one neuron run in bundles together with terminal fibers of other neurons. Thus, each adrenergic fiber innervates many effector cells and each effector cell is innervated by many adrenergic fibers which originate from different neurons. The average total length of the terminal

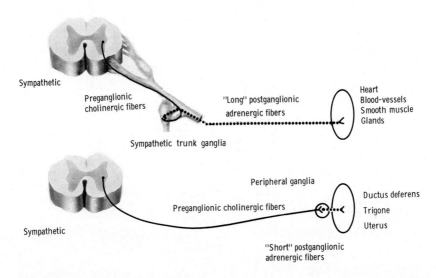

Figure 25. Schematic representation of two systems of adrenergic neurons. There are two systems of adrenergic neurons: one "long" and the other "short." The long adrenergic neurons have their cell bodies located in the paravertebral and prevertebral sympathetic ganglia and innervate smooth muscle and glands in many peripheral tissues. The short adrenergic neurons have their cell bodies located in ganglia close to or within the pelvic organs of the urinogenital tract. From these ganglia short adrenergic axons originate which innervate accessory male genital organs, urethra, parts of the female reproductive tract and the trigonal area of the urinary bladder.

system of each neuron is about 10 cm. These ramifications of the axons are true terminals. They often form basket-like arrangements around the innervated components. On these terminals, at regular intervals, are bead-like structures called varicosities (Fig. 26) which are believed to be presynaptic

SCHEMATIC REPRESENTATION OF NERVE ENDING AND DENSE CORE VESICLES (STORAGE SITE FOR CATECHOLAMINE) IN A SYMPATHETIC NEURON.

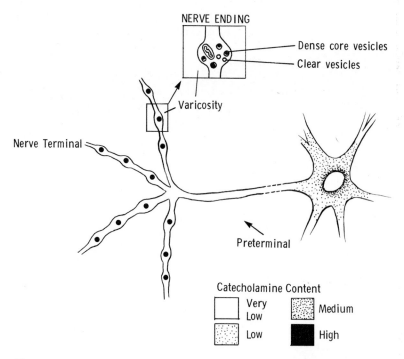

Figure 26. Schematic representation of adrenergic neuron showing cell body, the preterminal axon and nerve terminal network.

When the axon approaches the tissue to be innervated, it becomes varicose. In the innervated tissue, each axon splits into a system of branches called nerve terminals. As the axon enters the smooth muscle, its diameter alternately increases and decreases every few microns, giving the axon a beaded appearance. These bead-like structures are called varicosites. The release of the neurotransmitter is believed to occur from these varicose enlargements, where the neurotransmitter is stored in high concentration in storage particles. Under normal conditions, the terminal region may contain three times the amount of the transmitter found in the cell body.

structures from which norepinephrine is released in response to a nerve stimulus.

The varicosities are about 1 to 2 μ in diameter and are separated from one another by about 3 μ. Studies based on histochemical fluorescence methods have shown that nerve cell bodies have a low catecholamine content and that practically the total amount of the adrenergic transmitter is localized in the varicosities of synaptic terminals. The ratio between the norepinephrine content of cell bodies and of terminals is calculated to be 1 : 300. Each varicosity contains about 0.005 Pg (picograms) of norepinephrine and the number of varicosities per neuron is about 26,000. The varicosities contain dense groups of small membrane-bound particles. In electron micrographs these particles are seen to be distributed in the axoplasm of the nerve fiber together with some other intracellular organelles such as mitochondria.

Studies with the electron microscope show that cholinergic, like adrenergic nerve terminals in smooth muscle possess varicosities. It is, therefore, likely that the terminal apparatus of a cholinergic axon is similar to that of an adrenergic axon.

Innervation of Blood Vessels

In contrast to the smooth muscle in other viscera, the nerve terminals in the smooth muscle of blood vessels are not distributed throughout the muscle layers. Adrenergic fibers ramify extensively in the adventitia of most blood vessels. In elastic arteries, adrenergic terminals are confined to the adventitia whereas in muscular arteries and arterioles vasomotor fibers approach the media but rarely penetrate beyond its outer layer. The vasomotor activity in these vessels, therefore, is neurogenic in the case of the outer smooth muscle layers and myogenic in the inner layers.

In cutaneous veins which are relatively thick-walled, many adrenergic fibers are in the media, whereas veins in skeletal muscles have relatively few fibers in the media.

Vasomotor neuromuscular junctions are characterized by considerably large synaptic clefts (60–400 Å). The nerve-muscle relationship becomes closer as the vessel size diminishes so that in terminal arterioles, precapillary sphincters and venules there is a relatively close contact between axons and muscle cells.

Some blood vessels are innervated by cholinergic nerve fibers, e.g. skeletal muscle vessels. The cholinergic innervation, like the adrenergic, is confined to the adventitial-media junction of the vessel wall.

SYNAPTIC VESICLES

One of the main characteristics of nerve terminals with chemical synapses is the presence of spherical organelles about 50 nm in diameter called synaptic vesicles. At the motor end-plate these vesicles are aggregated at sites on the nerve terminal membrane and are concerned with the release of acetylcholine in response to nerve stimulation.

Synaptic vesicles are present within the varicosities of both adrenergic and cholinergic postganglionic nerve terminals.

Adrenergic Vesicles

Electron microscopic and biochemical studies show that the size of the vesicles varies in different parts of the adrenergic neuron. In the nerve terminal the vesicles are mainly of small size, with only a small percentage being the large type. In the cell body and in the axon, vesicles are mainly of large size. Large vesicles are all granular, whereas the small vesicles are of two types, granular and agranular. Granular vesicles contain a core of electron dense material. Norepinephrine is stored in the granular vesicles. Injected intravenously, norepinephrine is localized by electron microscopic autoradiography within the granular vesicles of sympathetic nerves. When an adrenergic nerve is ligated, proximal to the constriction there is an accumulation of granular vesicles significantly larger and more completely granulated than those found in the terminals.

Since the concentration of norepinephrine in sympathetic neurons can be correlated with the presence of larger as well as smaller granular vesicles, it is possible that the larger, more granular vesicles which occur in perikarya and preterminal axons may be the precursor of the synaptic vesicles. These larger vesicles are synthesized in the cell body and are transported to the axon terminals where they are transformed into small synaptic vesicles. Thus, in the terminal varicosities there are three types of vesicles: large dense core vesicles (600 to 1500 Å); small dense core vesicles (300 to 600 Å); and small agranular vesicles (300 to 600 Å). The small vesicles are the predominent type in the varicosities.

Whereas dense core vesicles are the site of synthesis, storage and release of norepinephrine, the function and significance of agranular vesicles is far from clear.

CONTENTS OF VESICLES. The granular vesicles contain, in addition to catecholamines, large amounts of adenine nucleotide (primarily adenosine triphosphate, ATP). The molar ratio of catecholamines to ATP is approximately 4 : 1. The vesicles also contain large amounts of soluble protein (1.8 mg/mg catecholamine). The majority of these proteins are nonenzymic although soluble dopamine-β-oxidase is also present. The soluble proteins have been fractionated into eight proteins and have been named collectively chromogranins. The chromogranins include one major (30 to 40%) soluble protein, chromogranin A. When an adrenergic axon is ligated, dopamine-β-oxidase and catecholamine-binding proteins accumulate proximal to the axonal con-

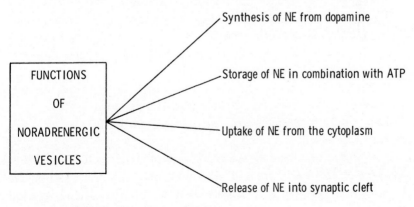

Figure 27.

striction, in a fashion similar to norepinephrine and its granular vesicles. These findings suggest that the site of synthesis of these proteins is in the soma of the neuron. Once formed, the proteins are transported into the axon terminals and incorporated into vesicles within the axons, either as components of the granular vesicles or else separately, perhaps by the neurotubules. What function some of the proteins from catecholamine vesicles serve is not clear. They may serve solely to bind the transmitter within vesicles until the moment of release.

FUNCTION OF STORAGE VESICLES (Fig. 27).

1. The dense core vesicles contain the enzyme dopamine-β-hydroxylase. They take up dopamine from the cytoplasm of the neuron and oxidize it to norepinephrine.
2. They store norepinephrine and maintain its levels by synthesis. Norepinephrine is stored in these particles in combination with adenosine triphosphate (ATP). The molar ratio of norepinephrine to ATP is 4 : 1. Binding of norepinephrine retards its diffusion out of the cell thereby protecting it from enzymatic destruction by the enzyme monoamine oxidase which is present in the cytoplasm of the neuron. The storage of norepinephrine in the granules is not specific because these granules can retain other structurally related compounds such as octopamine, α-methyl norepinephrine and metaraminol.
3. These vesicles take up norepinephrine from the adjacent cytoplasm after the transmitter has been recaptured by the neuronal cell membrane. The uptake process appears to require ATP and Mg^{++}.
4. These vesicles are the site from which norepinephrine and protein are released directly into the synaptic cleft.

Thus, storage vesicles are the site of synthesis, storage, and release of norepinephrine.

SYNTHESIS AND TRANSPORT OF VESICLES. It is well known that ligation of the axon prevents the flow of a material within the axoplasm to the nerve terminals. Within minutes of the ligation of a rat sympathetic nerve, norepinephrine accumulates above the ligation. As the constriction is moved closer and closer toward, and finally within the ganglia, the accumulation of norepinephrine within the granules is seen above each level of constriction. The accumulation of norepinephrine is clearly seen in the ganglia and can be followed into the perikarya. This accumulation of norepinephrine is abolished by reserpine which is known to deplete norepinephrine. These observations suggest that the accumulated granules are formed in the perikarya, and that there is a proximo-distal transport of these amine-containing granules. The ultrastructural details of the granular vesicles indicate that most of the granular vesicles that accumulated in or above the constriction were larger than the majority of the granular vesicles in the adrenergic terminals. On the basis of this type of experiment, it has been suggested that the large dense core vesicles are synthesized in the cell body of the neuron and are transported to the axon terminals. These may serve as precursors of the synaptic vesicles.

Life Span of the Granules. According to Dahlström and Haggendal, the life span of the amine granules is three to four weeks which relates to their ability to retain endogenous norepinephrine. However, the properties of young, newly formed granules change with age.

Life Cycle of Storage Vesicles.

1. Chromogranins are synthesized by ribosomes of the endoplasmic reticulum in the soma of the adrenergic neuron.
2. They are transferred to the Golgi apparatus, where they are encased in membrane-limited vesicles.
3. These vesicles are transported rapidly down the axon into its varicose terminals.
4. At varicose terminals they are stored in the varicosities.
5. Large vesicles are transformed into smaller vesicles.
6. This transformation may be followed by a process of exocytosis.

Cholinergic Vesicles

Electron microscopic studies at cholinergic nerve terminals indicate that the great majority of vesicles are small and agranular; the remainder are large and granular. There are no small granular vesicles at cholinergic nerve terminals. The diameter of the small agranular vesicle is about 45 nm. These vesicles take up and store acetylcholine and accumulation occurs against a concentration gradient.

The synaptic vesicles in cholinergic nerves are believed to be manufactured in the cell body and are transported distally along the axon as in adrenergic nerves. However, it is possible that some vesicles may be synthesized in the nerve terminal from neurotubules.

CHAPTER 6

RELEASE OF NEUROTRANSMITTERS

Spontaneous Release

T HE DISTINCTIVE FEATURE OF chemical transmission at synapses is the release of transmitter at nerve terminals. Nerve terminals release small amounts of transmitter into the synaptic cleft at random intervals in the absence of any nerve impulse. This spontaneous random discharge of neurotransmitter occurs in fairly uniform packets termed "quanta" consisting of many thousands of molecules. Each quantum corresponds to the amount of transmitter in one synaptic vesicle. The vesicle usually ruptures and discharges its content into the synaptic cleft. The released transmitter diffuses across the synaptic cleft and acts on specific receptor sites on the postsynaptic membrane to evoke postsynaptic potentials. These potentials, however, are too small to produce any activity in the effector cell and are termed "miniature potentials."

Spontaneous "miniature potentials" were first noticed by Fat and Katz as early as 1950 in frog neuromuscular junctions. They found highly localized activity consisting of small depolarizations occurring intermittently at random intervals with an average frequency of about one per second at the end-plate region. These miniature potentials have the same characteristics as end-plate potentials neurally evoked except for their spon-

79

taneous occurrence and small amplitude. Their time course, localization and response to various agents which modify the action of transmitter is similar to end-plate potentials evoked by nerve impulses.

Spontaneous miniature potentials have been observed at all chemical transmitting synapses, both peripheral and central, as well as excitatory and inhibitory. They have the following general characteristics:

1. The amplitudes of spontaneous miniature potentials show little variation about the mean. There is an occasional occurrence of a potential whose amplitude is a multiple of the mean. It thus appears that quantal release is roughly of the same magnitude. Inhibition of synthesis of neurotransmitter may lead to reduction of transmitter content of each quanta which correspondingly diminishes the mean miniature potential during nerve stimulation.

2. Miniature junction potentials have the appropriate polarization, that is, they cause depolarization at excitatory synapses and hyperpolarization at inhibitory synapses.

3. The amplitude is not the same on all synapses; variation in amplitude of miniature junction potentials from synapse to synapse may be due to variation in sensitivity of receptors on the effector cell rather than variation in the amount of the transmitter released.

4. Changes in Ca^{++} concentration in the extracellular medium cause relatively small alterations in the frequencies of the spontaneous miniature potentials.

5. The average frequency of occurrence of spontaneous miniature junction potentials is sensitive to presynaptic potentials, osmotic pressure differences across the cell membrane, and temperature. A striking increase in frequency of release of miniature potentials is observed with increases in temperature, osmotic pressure, and depolarizing potentials. These factors neither affect significantly the transmitter content of each packet nor their mean amplitude. These factors may affect the "activation barrier" and thereby increase the probability of random release.

Release of Transmitter by a Nerve Impulse

The arrival of a conducted nerve impulse leads to a synchronus discharge of many quanta within less than one millisecond, thereby generating an end-plate potential. Usually 500 to 1000 molecules of transmitter are released per impulse at a single synapse. The quantum of the transmitter release remains unchanged whether it occurs spontaneously during the period of rest or at the peak of the activity of the axon membrane when the impulse arrives at the nerve terminal. Thus it appears that the normal end-plate potential is generated following nerve stimulation by the synchronous release of quanta of the transmitter, the individual spontaneous liberation of which gives rise to a miniature potential. Quanta release continues even when nerve terminal membranes are completely depolarized. The features of neurotransmitter release are summarized in Figure 28.

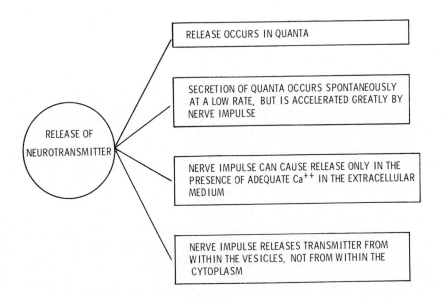

Figure 28.

Role of Calcium

When an action potential travelling along a nerve fiber reaches the nerve terminals, a sequence of events is initiated that results in the release of a transmitter. An influx of calcium is essential for a quantal transmitter release. It is believed that depolarization of the nerve terminal increases its membrane permeability to calcium; calcium enters the terminal and, after a variable delay, release of the transmitter occurs.

The release of acetylcholine, norepinephrine, and epinephrine upon stimulation of their respective synapses is prevented in the absence of Ca^{++}. In the perfused suprarenal gland it has been observed that the amount of catecholamine released in response to splanchnic nerve stimulation depends on the concentration of Ca^{++} in the perfusing fluid, being greater when the Ca^{++} is greater. It seems that the presence of Ca^{++} is a general requirement of chemical synapses. The relationship between the extracellular concentration of Ca^{++} and transmitter release is not always linear.

Spontaneous secretion is not abolished in the absence of Ca^{++}. At cholinergic synapses a basal resting secretion of acetylcholine is reduced in the absence of Ca^{++}, whereas at adrenergic synapses spontaneous release may increase.

Magnesium, which is predominantly an intracellular cation has an action opposite that of calcium. When present in the extracellular medium, magnesium competes with calcium for the action sites and depresses the release of transmitter in response to nerve stimulation. An increase in the Ca^{++} concentration partially overcomes the effects of increased Mg^{++}. The role of ions in the release of neurotransmitters has not been fully elucidated as yet.

Regulation of Transmitter Release through a Negative Feedback Mechanism

Recent reports from a number of laboratories suggest that the release of a transmitter as a result of stimulation of the nerve terminal is regulated by a negative feedback mechanism. According to this theory, a neurotransmitter released in response to a nerve impulse, may inhibit the additional release of neurotransmitter in response to subsequent impulses due to a sufficient concentration of transmitter substance in the synaptic cleft.

In the perfused rabbit-heart preparation, stimulation of sympathetic nerves leads to the appearance of norepinephrine in the venous fluid leaving the heart. When an alpha-receptor blocking agent such as phenoxybenzamine or phentolamine is added to the perfusing fluid, the release of norepinephrine in response to nerve stimulation is greatly enhanced. The increased release of neurotransmitter after administering alpha-blocking agents occurs at concentrations that neither alter the uptake of amine across the neuronal membrane nor block the activation of norepinephrine at the neuroeffector junction.

In tissues pre-incubated with labelled norepinephrine, the total counts in the overflow during nerve stimulation are greatly increased after alpha-blocking drugs. This indicates that alpha-blocking drugs cause the release of more neurotransmitter than is normally released from the nerve terminals per nerve impulse. The release of norepinephrine in response to nerve stimulation is accompanied by the release of other components of granules such as dopamine-β-oxidase. Alpha-blocking agents not only increase the release of norepinephrine in response to nerve stimulation, but also increase the release of dopamine-β-oxidase. All these findings indicate that in the presence of alpha-blocking drugs, the increase in neurally-evoked release is not due to any alteration in inactivating mechanisms at the nerve terminal-effector cell level, but rather is due to the increased release from the amine granules in the nerve terminal.

In the perfused rabbit heart, the addition of norepinephrine in the perfusing medium diminishes the secretion of norepinephrine induced by stimulation of sympathetic nerves. Alpha-blocking agents antagonize the inhibitory effect of exogenous norepinephrine.

From all of these findings the following theory has been deduced. In the vicinity of adrenergic nerve terminals, there may exist some receptors which modulate the release of norepinephrine induced by nerve stimulation. Activation of these receptors by norepinephrine (exogenous or released) decreases the average transmitter quantum discharged per nerve impulse, whereas blockade of these receptors by alpha-blocking drugs increases the release of neurotransmitter. Thus, the release of norepinephrine by nerve impulses is feedback inhibited; released norepinephrine and receptors sensitive to alpha-blocking agents are links in this feedback mechanism.

Some investigators have termed these receptors as alpha-receptors since they are blocked by alpha-blocking drugs. However, these alpha-receptors may differ from the alpha-adrenergic receptors which are located in the postsynaptic sites and mediate the response of the effector organs.

A negative feedback mechanism for acetylcholine released by nerve stimulation, similar to the one described for norepinephrine, has also been suggested. It has been found that cholinesterase inhibitors, which prevent the hydrolysis of released acetylcholine, inhibit the neurally evoked release of acetylcholine. It appears that cholinesterase inhibitors, by preventing hydrolysis of released acetylcholine, cause accumulation of the transmitter in the synaptic cleft. This in turn may act to inhibit the further release of cholinesterase inhibitors. The inhibition of acetylcholine release by a cholinesterase inhibitor is reversed by atropine which blocks muscarinic receptors. Thus

---

Figure 29. Schematic representation of negative feedback mechanism for the regulation of transmitter during nerve stimulation.

Release of transmitter in response to nerve stimulation is regulated by a negative feedback mechanism. Accordingly, the released transmitter may inhibit its own release once threshold concentration is achieved in the synaptic cleft. Some receptors or receptor-like structures in the vicinity of the nerve terminal are involved in a local feedback regulation of transmitter release. Stimulation of these receptors by the released transmitter may inhibit further release of transmitters during nerve stimulation whereas blockade of these receptors increases the release of the neurotransmitters. Release of transmitter activates the receptor and thereby depresses the secretory response to further arriving nerve impulses. ⟶

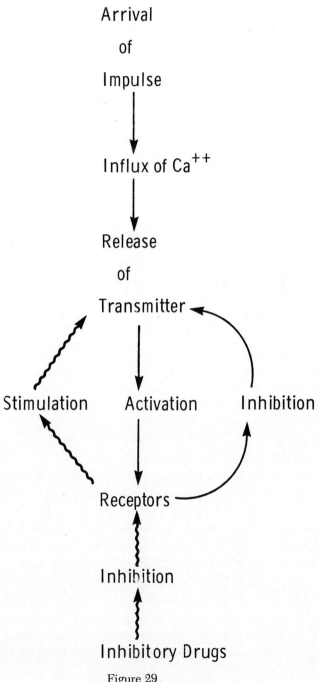

Figure 29.

it appears that at cholinergic synapses, acetylcholine regulates its own release per nerve impulse, and this feedback inhibition is mediated through muscarinic receptors.

Therefore, it seems that the existence of feedback mechanisms which regulate the release of neurotransmitters is a general phenomenon and occurs not only for norepinephrine but for acetylcholine as well (Fig. 29).

Release of Norepinephrine

The view generally held is that the impulse which passes along the sympathetic postganglionic fiber makes the membrane of the fiber permeable to calcium ions from the extracellular fluid. This entry of calcium ions causes, in some unknown way, the release of norepinephrine (Fig. 30).

Burn suggested that there is a cholinergic link in the release of norepinephrine. The hypothesis states that the impulse passing down the fiber first releases acetylcholine. This acetylcholine, probably after leaving the fibers, makes the membrane more permeable to calcium ions. These ions enter the fibers and release norepinephrine from the granules (Fig. 31).

Both these hypotheses have one common denominator in that the release of norepinephrine involves the inflow of calcium ions. The difference between them lies in the events between the action potential and the influx of calcium ions.

Exocytosis

The mechanism of release of catecholamines involves a process of exocytosis (*see* Structure 1). Exocytosis implies release of stored secretory products to the cell exterior without loss of cytoplasmic constituents. The release of catecholamines is thus accompanied by the release of all other components of the granules: adenine nucleotides, chromogranins, and the soluble portions of dopamine-β-oxidase. Each of the components released is directly proportional to the catecholamines as they occur in the intact storage vesicles.

This release does not, however, involve the extrusion of entire vesicles because vesicular membranes are not discharged, but remain in the cell as discrete structures. Since half of the dopamine-β-oxidase activity is present in the insoluble form associated with the vesicular membrane, stimulation of the suprarenal medulla leads to a release of the soluble portion of the enzyme only from the vesicles. Stimulation does not decrease the quantity of membrane-bound enzymes. Since after release norepinephrine, but not dopamine-β-oxidase, is rapidly inactivated, it is possible that circulating levels of dopamine-β-oxidase might constitute a better index of sympathetic function in the intact organism than the assay of neurotransmitter itself.

Whereas the components of granules are released, the macromolecules present in the cytoplasm of the neuron are not released during nerve stimulation. For example, tyrosine hydroxylase, which is a cytoplasmic enzyme, is not released during the exocytosis process. Likewise, phenyl-ethanolamine-N-methyl transferase (PNMT) present in the chromaffin cell cytoplasm is not secreted from the perfused suprarenal medulla during stimulation.

Various Types of Release of Norepinephrine

Four different types of release seem to occur:

1. *Resting Secretion.* There is strong evidence that the effector organ is normally under the influence of a "resting secretion" of norepinephrine from postganglionic sympathetic nerves comparable to the resting secretion of the suprarenal medulla. This resting secretion may be visualized as consisting of two components (a) spontaneous random discharge of packets or quanta of norepinephrine to set up the so-called miniature junction potentials in the effector cells. However, the amount of norepinephrine so released is far too small to cause a mechanical response of the effector organ and (b) release of relatively large amounts of norepinephrine as a result of impulse traffic from the central nervous system, for the purpose of maintaining tonic activity particularly in the vascular smooth muscle.

2. *Release of Norepinephrine by the Nerve Impulse* (*Fig. 32*). The arrival of a conducted nerve impulse leads to the discharge of many quanta, and thus causes a mechanical re-

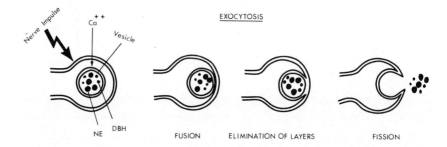

Structure 1. *A possible mechanism of release of catecholamines by exocytosis.* Catecholamines (CA) are released from the nerve terminals. In the case of the adrenal medulla and postganglionic sympathetic nerve endings, the mechanism of release of CA involves a process of exocytosis, whereby the entire soluble content of the vesicles are discharged to the exterior of the cell. On the arrival of an impulse, the nerve is depolarized and the storage vesicles fuse with the inner membrane of the nerve terminal; this is followed by the formation of an opening large enough to extrude the entire soluble content of the vesicles. Thus, the release of CA is accompanied by the release of all other soluble components of granules: adenine nucleotide (ATP), chromogranin and the soluble portion of dopamine-B-hydroxylase (DBH). The vesicular membranes are not discharged, but remain in the cell as discrete structures. The exocytotic process requires the presence of CA^{++}. There might be a contractile microfilament on the neuronal membrane which is activated by CA^{++} thus making an opening for the discharge of the soluble contents of the vesicle.

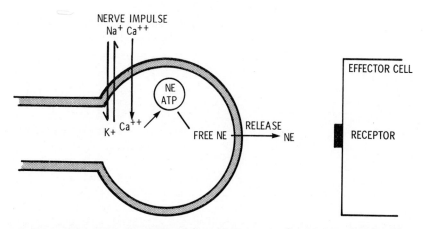

Figure 30. Schematic representation of the events leading to the release of norepinephrine. The arrival of the nerve impulse in the adrenergic nerve terminals causes a series of changes of the ionic permeability of the cell membrane and permits the entry of calcium ions from the extracellular fluid. This entry of calcium ions causes, in some unknown way, the release of norepinephrine.

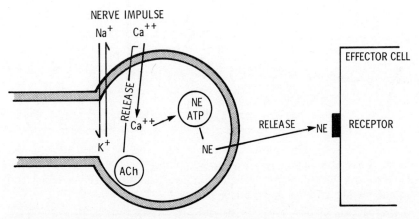

Figure 31. Schematic representation of the release of norepinephrine from adrenergic nerve terminals according to the cholinergic-link theory. The impulse in the adrenergic nerve terminals first releases acetylcholine. The acetylcholine probably leaves the fibers and acts on the nerve cell membrane, changing its permeability to calcium ions. The entry of the calcium ions then causes the release of norepinephrine from the storage granules.

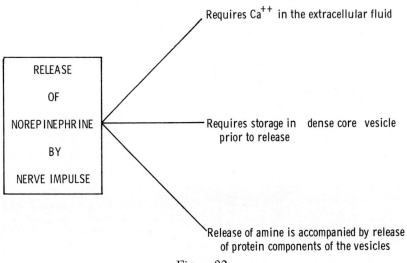

Figure 32.

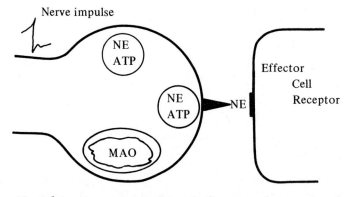

Figure 33. Schematic representation of the site of nerve-impulse release. Nerve stimulation releases norepinephrine from the storage vesicles close to the synaptic cleft. Norepinephrine leaves the nerve terminal and is not metabolized by monoamine oxidase.

Figure 35. Schematic representation of the site of action of reserpine or guanethidine in the adrenergic neuron. Reserpine and guanethidine act on vesicles which are more deeply located in the neuron. The released norepinephrine is exposed to the action of monoamine oxidase. Thus norepinephrine leaves the nerve terminals as an inactivated deaminated metabolite. →

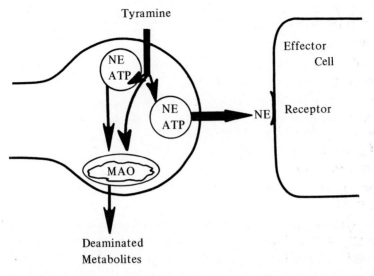

Figure 34. Schematic representation of the site of action of tyramine in the adrenergic neuron. Tyramine displaces the norepinephrine from its storage site. The release of norepinephrine from vesicles occurs throughout the cytoplasm of the nerve terminals both deep and close to the synaptic cleft. Some norepinephrine leaves the nerve terminals; however, substantial amounts of norepinephrine are oxidatively deaminated within the neuron. Tyramine itself is a good substrate for monoamine oxidase and part of the injected amine is destroyed by the monoamine oxidase.

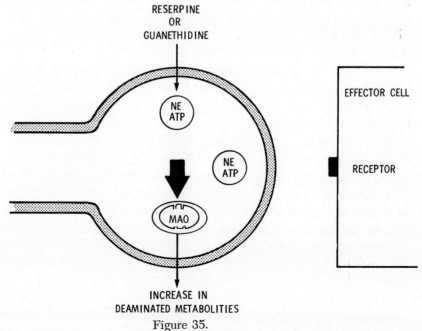

Figure 35.

sponse in the effector organ. It has been estimated that 500 to 1000 molecules of transmitter are released per impulse at a single synapse. Nerve stimulation appears to release norepinephrine more directly and rapidly into the extraneuronal spaces. De Robertis and Ferreira have suggested that during nerve stimulation norepinephrine is released from vesicles located immediately adjacent to the cell membrane at the neuron (Fig. 33). ATP is lost, together with stored amine.

Catecholamine in the cytoplasm is not released by nerve stimulation, suggesting that transmitter has to be incorporated into the storage granules before it can be released by nerve impulses.

3. *Release of Norepinephrine by Tyramine-like Drugs.* Indirectly acting amines such as tyramine and amphetamine displace the transmitter from the storage site. This type of release is not acccompanied by a loss of ATP from the granules, and there is mole-by-mole substitution of tyramine molecule for the bound norepinephrine. Substantial amounts of norepinephrine released by the indirectly acting amine are oxidatively deaminated within the nerve terminal.

While nerve stimulation releases norepinephrine directly into the synaptic cleft, an indirectly acting amine (tyramine, amphetamine) apparently releases norepinephrine from vesicles throughout the cytoplasm of the nerve terminal at such a rate that appreciable amounts are oxidatively deaminated before leaving the nerve terminal (Fig. 34).

4. *Release of Norepinephrine by Reserpine.* Reserpine releases large amounts of norepinephrine, but it produces little physiological effect. Reserpine causes a slow release of norepinephrine presumably from vesicles which are deep in the neuron (Fig. 35). The released norepinephrine is exposed to the action of monoamine oxidase in the mitochondria present in the nerves. Thus, norepinephrine leaves the nerve terminals as an inactive deaminated metabolite. Guanethidine resembles reserpine insofar as it causes depletion of peripheral norepinephrine stores. ATP may be lost together with stored amine.

CHAPTER 7

SYNTHESIS AND
INACTIVATION OF TRANSMITTERS

ACETYLCHOLINE

ACETYLCHOLINE is a neurotransmitter at cholinergic nerve endings and is an acetic acid ester of choline (FIG. 36).

Synthesis

Synthesis of acetylcholine (ACh) takes place in nerve endings and requires choline (precursor), choline acetylase, and acetyl coenzyme A. The choline required for transmitter synthesis is provided by an extracellular source. It is taken up by the nerve terminal. Hemicholinium compounds block uptake of choline by the nerve terminal and thereby interfere with the synthesis of acetylcholine.

The distribution of choline acetylase closely parallels that of acetylcholine. Both are present in high concentration in cholinergic nerves. They disappear rapidly when these nerves are cut and time is allowed for them to degenerate. Hebb and Waites presented evidence that the enzyme choline acetylase is formed in the soma and is transported to the endings by axoplasmic flow. In nerve terminals it is present outside of the synaptic vesicles as well as in the vesicles. It is uncertain

93

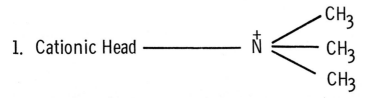

1. Cationic Head ——————— $\overset{+}{N}$ $\begin{cases} CH_3 \\ CH_3 \\ CH_3 \end{cases}$

2. Two Carbon Chains Which
   Link Cationic Head With an ——— $CH_2\text{-}CH_2$
   Ester Group

3. Ester Group ——————— $O — C — CH_3$
   $\quad\quad\quad\quad\quad\quad\quad\quad\quad\quad\quad\quad\quad\quad\quad \| $
   $\quad\quad\quad\quad\quad\quad\quad\quad\quad\quad\quad\quad\quad\quad\quad O$

Figure 36. Features of acetylcholine molecule.

whether acetylcholine is synthesized in the synaptic vesicles or whether it is only stored there after it has been synthesized elsewhere. The occurrence of choline acetylase has been used for identifying sites of acetylcholine synthesis. Therefore, it is possible that some synthesis occurs outside the vesicle and some in conjunction with synaptic vesicles.

Coenzyme A and choline are widely distributed and found in most tissues.

Two steps are involved in the synthesis of acetylcholine. In the first stage, acetyl coenzyme A is formed from acetate in the presence of the "acetate-activating" enzyme acetylkinase.

Activation of acetate coenzyme A ——→ acetyl coenzyme A

The second stage involves the transfer of the acetyl group from acetyl coenzyme A to choline. The action is catalyzed by the enzyme choline acetylase:

aectyl coenzyme A + choline choline acetylase → acetylcholine
+ coenzyme A

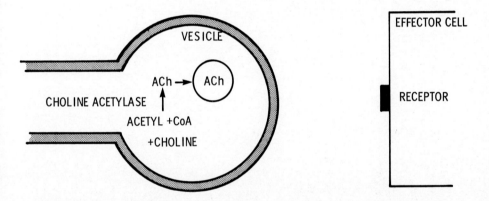

Figure 37. The synthesis of acetylocholine. Synthesis of acetylcholine by choline acetylase takes place in the cytoplasm. It is then stored in synaptic vesicles.

STEP   I   Formation of Complex

Ach + Enzyme $\rightleftharpoons$ Ach-Enzyme
                                                   Complex

STEP II   Liberation of Choline

Ach-Enzyme $\longrightarrow$ Acetylated Enzyme
     Complex   +
                                                  Choline

STEP iII   Regeneration of Enzyme

$$\text{Acetylated Enzyme} \xrightarrow{\text{H}_2\text{O}} \text{Enzyme + Acetic Acid}$$

Figure 38. Hydrolysis of acetylcholine.

The major energy source of this reaction is adenosine triphosphate (ATP). Sodium ions are necessary for optimal synthesis. The synthesis is depicted in Figure 37.

During physiological activity, much more acetylcholine is released from the nerve terminals of a cholinergic neuron than is normally present in the resting neuron. These findings suggest that the rate of synthesis is increased during nerve stimulation to replenish the transmitter stores. The mechanism regulating acetylcholine synthesis is unclear. It is possible that a process of end-product inhibition occurs whereby the concentration of acetylcholine in the nerve terminal regulates its own rate of synthesis, because *in vitro* studies have shown that the activity of choline acetylase is inhibited by acetylcholine.

Hydrolysis

The hydrolysis of acetylcholine (ACh) takes place in three stages. The first stage involves the acetylcholine enzyme complex. This occurs because cholinesterase (AChE) has an active site which attracts acetylcholine. Nachmansohn has investigated the active site of cholinesterase and has suggested two subsites on the enzyme (Fig. 39). One of these is an anionic site which is chiefly concerned with specificity and is negatively charged. It attracts the positively charged nitrogen atom of acetylcholine (see Figs. 38, 40). This cationic head is absorbed into the anionic site of cholinesterase and forms a salt. The second is the esteratic site which contains a group G that may be an imidazole group and is concerned with the hydrolytic process. It is combined with a carbonyl C atom of the ester group. Acetylcholine is adsorbed on the enzyme to form an enzyme-substrate complex. The manner in which adsorption takes place has not been fully elucidated.

The second stage of hydrolysis involves splitting. The enzyme substrate complex reacts to release choline and leaves an acetylated enzyme. The released acetylcholine is taken up by the nerve terminal and is reused for acetylcholine synthesis. Thus, wherever acetylcholine is present to activate nerve tissue in order to effect transmission of the nerve impulse, AChE is there to hydrolyze it and terminate its action.

The third stage of hydrolysis is the regeneration of the enzyme. The acetylated enzyme reacts with water to give acetic acid and the enzyme, and thus the enzyme is regenerated (see Figs. 38, 40).

Anticholinesterase, as a physostigmine type molecule, enters into competitive displacement with ACh for the surface site in concentration as low as 15^6 M. Displacement by physostigmine prevents the enzyme to hydrolyze acetylcholine.

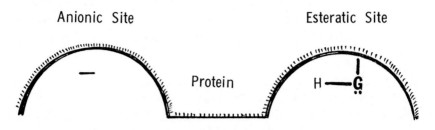

Figure 39.

Acetylcholinesterase (AChE)

The enzyme involved in the hydrolysis of acetylcholine is called acetylcholinesterase. Various types of esterases are found in animal tissue, but at least two show some degree of specificity for choline esters. There is a good correlation between the distribution of acetylcholinesterase, acetylcholine, and choline acetylase. The properties of both esterases are summarized in Table VIII.

Location

Histochemical studies indicate the presence of intracellular acetylcholinesterase. Acetylcholinesterase is also present external to the cell membrane of autonomic neurons. It is this external or functional acetylcholinesterase that is thought to be concerned with enzymatic destruction of the acetylcholine released from the terminals of the presynaptic fibers. At the neuromuscular junction, acetylcholinesterase is found external to both the presynaptic and postsynaptic elements. The major events at a typical cholinergic synapse are presented in Figure 41.

NOREPINEPHRINE

Biosynthesis

Catecholamines are synthesized in peripheral and central adrenergic neurons and in the chromaffin cells of the suprarenal medulla. Synthesis of catecholamines is a complex process; it

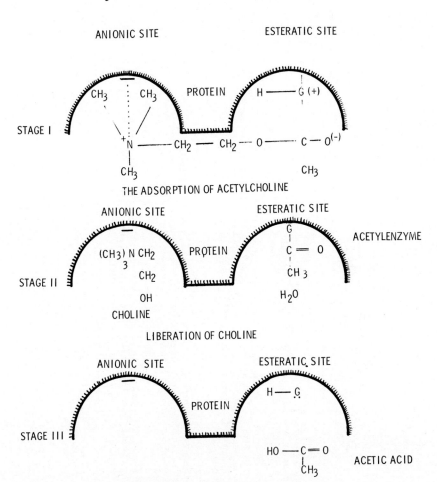

Figure 40. Regeneration of enzyme.

proceeds as follows: tyrosine ⟶ dopa-dopamine ⟶ norepinephrine-epinephrine. The natural precursor is l-tyrosine which is present in the circulation in the amount of about 15 mg per liter. It is taken up by adrenergic neurons. The nature and kinetics of tyrosine transport into the neuron are not known completely. Once inside the neuron, tyrosine is converted to dopa by the enzyme tyrosine hydroxylase. The enzyme is specific for l-tyrosine and requires oxygen, iron, and a tetrahy-

TABLE VIII
CHOLINESTERASE

	true	pseudo
Occurrence:	1. Red blood cell 2. Nervous system 3. Human placenta	1. Blood serum 2. Intestine 3. Skin and many other tissues
Specificity:	High affinity for ACh rate of substrate hydrolysis decreases with an increase in length of acyl chain: acetyl> proprionyl> butyrylcholine	Weaker affinity for ACh; rate of hydrolysis increases with an increase in length of chain: butyryl> propionyl> acetylcholine
Substrate concentration:	*Optimal:* rate of hydrolysis is maximum only at optimal concentration (decreases for weaker or stronger solution)	*Not optimal:* rate of hydrolysis increases with increase in substrate concentration
Function:	ACh released endogenously is mostly hydrolyzed by true ChE	Function is uncertain except in the intestine where it may control the activity of ACh

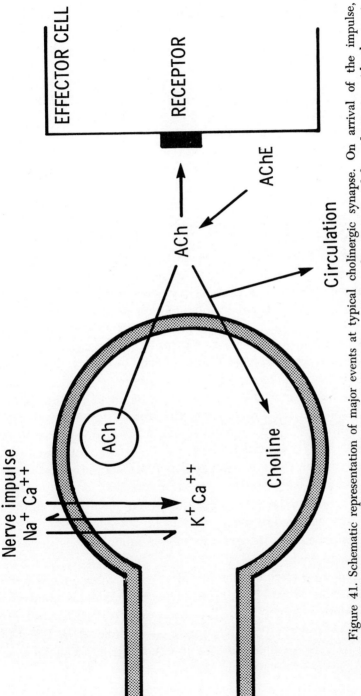

Figure 41. Schematic representation of major events at typical cholinergic synapse. On arrival of the impulse, acetylcholine is released from synaptic vesicles. It diffuses across the synaptic cleft and reacts with the post-synaptic membrane. The mechanism of release by nerve impulses is not certain: it does require Ca^{++}. On hydrolysis, choline is released into circulation and some may be taken up by the pre-synaptic synthetic sites.

dropteridine cofactor for its optimal activity. The enzyme is present in the brain, in the suprarenal medulla, and within adrenergic nervous tissue. Its exact location in the neuron is not known, but it appears to occur in the axoplasm of the nerve terminal. A variety of catecholamines including dopamine and norepinephrine inhibit the enzyme tyrosine hydroxylase by competing with the tetrahydropteridine cofactor. The relatively low activity of this enzyme makes it a rate-limiting enzyme in the biosynthesis of catecholamines.

Dopa is converted to dopamine by a dopa decarboxylase (*l*-aromatic amino acid decarboxylase). The enzyme requires pyridoxal phosphate as cofactor. This enzyme is relatively unspecific and is present in excess so that dopa does not accumulate, but is immediately converted to dopamine. These two enzymatically catalyzed reactions occur in the axoplasm of the nerve terminal. The dopamine is either destroyed by monoamine oxidase (an enzyme present in the cytoplasm of the neuron and associated with mitochondria) or taken up into the storage vesicle where it is converted to norepinephrine by the enzyme dopamine-β-oxidase. This reaction requires molecular oxygen, ascorbate, and enzyme-bound copper. This enzyme is entirely localized in the storage granules, so that dopamine must enter the granules in order to be hydroxylated. The transport of dopamine across the storage granules requires Mg^{++} and ATP, and can be blocked by a drug known as reserpine. The norepinephrine forms a stable complex with ATP and protein within the vesicles. Norepinephrine which is not bound may leak into the cytoplasm and may be deaminated by monoamine oxidase. The enzyme dopamine-β-oxidase is nonspecific and can hydroxylate a variety of phenylethylamines besides dopamine. The biosynthesis of norepinephrine is depicted in Figure 42.

The final step in the formation of catecholamine involves the N-methylation of norepinephrine. This conversion is catalyzed by phenylethanolamine-N-methyl transferase (PNMT) and occurs almost exclusively in the suprarenal medulla. PNMT is also present in very small quantities in other tissues. The enzyme is found in the soluble fraction after centrifugation of suprarenal homogenates and requires S-adenosyl methionine for transfer of the methyl group to the amino group of norepinephrine. It

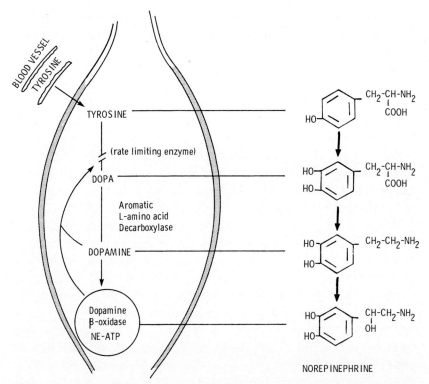

Figure 42. The biosynthesis of norepinephrine in an adrenergic neuron. The tyrosine is taken up from the plasma into the neuron and is subsequently hydroxylated to dopa by the enzyme tyrosine hydroxylase. The dopa is then decarboxylated in the cytoplasm by the enzyme L-aromatic amino acid decarboxylase. These two enzymatic catalyzed reactions take place in the cytoplasm of the neuron whereas conversion of dopamine to norepinephrine takes place only in the dense core vesicle. Apparently the dopamine is taken up into the dense core vesicle, where it is β-hydroxylated to norepinephrine by the enzyme dopamine β-oxidase. The dopamine which is not taken up is metabolized intraneuronally by monoamine oxidase. The levels of norepinephrine in the nerve are maintained by a negative feedback mechanism. The norepinephrine formed is stored in combination with ATP and perhaps other macromolecules of the vesicles.

is also nonspecific and can methylate a variety of β-phenyle-thanolamines. In the suprarenal medullary cell, norepinephrine migrates from chromaffin granules to the cytoplasm and is N-methylated to form epinephrine. Thus the pathway of catecholamine synthesis comprises three enzymes in the post-ganglionic sympathetic neurons and four in the suprarenal medulla.

Regulation of Synthesis

Physiological factors which control the rate of synthesis of norepinephrine in the adrenergic neurons are complex. Since endogenous levels of norepinephrine are maintained at a fixed level characteristic of each organ unless synthesis is inhibited, it appears that there is a dynamic balance between the rate of synthesis of norepinephrine and its disappearance.

When the splanchnic nerves to the suprarenal medulla are stimulated, there is a large increase in the catecholamine content of the venous effluent; however, there is little or no reduction in the catecholamine content of the medullary tissue. Likewise, increased sympathetic nerve activity causes little change in tissue catecholamine level. The maintenance of endogenous amine level is not possible, however, when norepinephrine synthesis is inhibited by the tyrosine hydroxylase inhibitor α-methyl p-tyrosine. In this case the catecholamine content is reduced significantly. Thus these findings suggest that catechol-amine synthesis is increased in response to sympathetic nerve stimulation in order to maintain normal levels of catecholamines in the organ.

Acceleration of norepinephrine synthesis due to nerve stimu-lation occurs at the tyrosine hydroxylation step because the rate of norepinephrine synthesis from tyrosine increases, whereas the rate of formation of norepinephrine from dopa and dopa-mine remains unaltered. The enhanced synthesis takes place without a significant change in tissue levels of tyrosine hy-droxylase. Norepinephrine and other catechols cause inhibition of the enzyme tyrosine hydroxylase. Accordingly, a pool of free catecholamines in the cytoplasm, in equilibrium with vesicular catecholamine, might regulate the tyrosine hydroxylase activity. Under normal conditions, tyrosine hydroxylase is apparently chronically inhibited by the free cytoplasmic levels of catecholamines. An increase in sympathetic nerve activity increases the efflux of norepinephrine and also in some way reduces the free cytoplasmic catecholamine concentration and thereby releases the tyrosine hydroxylase from end-product inhibition. The rate of conversion of tyrosine to dopa is enhanced. Conversely, if the activity of the sympathetic nervous system is reduced, free norepinephrine in the cytoplasm increases and inhibits the tyrosine hydroxylase activity. Thus this mechanism is capable of rapidly adjusting the rate of norepinephrine synthesis in response to changes in physiological demand for norepinephrine by altering the activity of tyrosine hydroxylase without affecting the amount of enzyme.

When increased sympathetic nerve activity is prolonged over a period of days, it provokes a long term adaptation which involves the induction of tyrosine hydroxylase and dopamine-β-oxidase. This induction is a slow process and it is neuronally mediated since it is abolished by prior denervation of the organ. The increase in catecholamine synthesizing enzyme activities is due to production of new enzyme protein rather than formation of an activator. It is abolished by cyclohexamide which inhibits protein synthesis at the translation level. Increased sympathetic nervous activity for a prolonged period of time also elevates the activities of dopamine-β-oxidase and PNMT.

Hormones can influence the activities of tyrosine hydroxylase, dopamine-β-oxidase and PNMT in the suprarenal gland. After removal of the pituitary gland, there is a gradual but marked diminution in activities of adrenal tyrosine hydroxylase, dopamine-β-oxidase and PNMT. Adrenocorticotropic hormone (ACTH) can restore activity of all these adrenal enzymes in hypophysectomized animals.

Thus two mechanisms seem to control catecholamine synthesis: one involving end-product inhibition of tyrosine hydroxylase and the other involving enzyme induction. Regulation of synthesis by end-product inhibition is rapid and the rate of synthesis of norepinephrine is adjusted immediately in response to changes in physiological demands for catecholamine. It is usually believed that only the intraneuronally unbound catecholamine is important in the feedback control of norepinephrine synthesis. An increase in sympathetic nerve activity, due to any stimulus, would increase the efflux of norepinephrine, and thereby could lower slightly the free intraneuronal cytoplasmic levels of the neurohormone. This decrease might diminish the end-product inhibition and thereby stimulate norepinephrine synthesis. On the other hand, procedures which either decrease the efflux of norepinephrine or which release norepinephrine from storage vesicles into cytoplasm, elicit an increase in free intraneuronal catecholamine and consequently an end-product inhibition of tyrosine hydroxylase occurs; this would exert an inhibitory effect on norepinephrine synthesis. It probably accounts for most of the regulation necessary to maintain the homeostasis.

The other mechanism, i.e. enzyme induction, in the control of norepinephrine synthesis, becomes effective only as a result of prolonged stimulation of the sympathetic nervous system. In this case, an increase in the rate of synthesis of norepinephrine is due to an increase in the synthesis and content of tyrosine hydoxylase and dopamine-β-oxidase. This process, however, is relatively slower.

Fate of Released Catecholamine

There is no enzyme similar to acetylcholinesterase at cholinergic synapses which can rapidly destroy catecholamines released at adrenergic synapses. Furthermore, the inactivation of catecholamines involves a number of processes and is not solely dependent on enzymatic degradation. The enzymes principally involved in the inactivation of norepinephrine or epinephrine are monoamine oxidase (MAO) and catechol-O-methyl transferase (COMT).

The catecholamines are almost entirely metabolized in the body, and only small quantities of unchanged amines are found in the urine. Metabolic degradation of catecholamines occurs by way of oxidative deamination and by O-methylation of the catechol nucleus. Mitochondrial monoamine oxidase is responsible for deamination, a pathway which is the predominant one in the neuron, but which also occurs extraneuronally. O-methy-

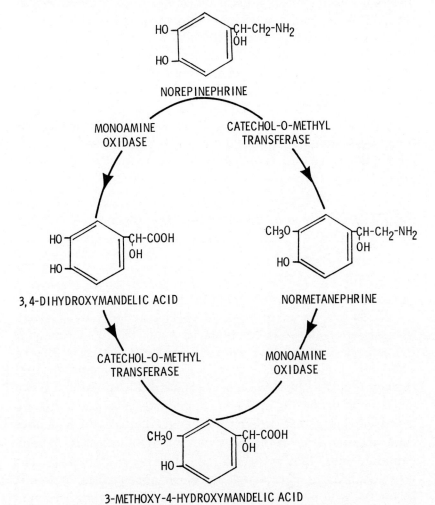

Figure 43. Metabolic pathway of norepinephrine.

lation by catechol-O-methyl-transferase, a soluble cytoplasmic enzyme, appears to be the dominant mechanism of degradation outside the neuron. Both the deaminated and O-methylated metabolites of the catecholamines are substrates for subsequent degradation by the alternate enzymes, and the final common metabolite is 3-methoxy-4-hydroxymandelic acid (vanilmandelic acid). This metabolic pathway is presented in Figure 43.

Although O-methylated metabolites, metanephrine, and normetanephrine represent a smaller fraction of the urinary metabolites of epinephrine and norepinephrine, they are a better measure of the quantity of amines released in a physiologically active form than are the deaminated products. The relative daily excretion of free catecholamines and of their metabolites is approximately: norepinephrine and epinephrine, 0.1 mg; normetanephrine and metanephrine, 1.3 mg; and vanilmandelic acid, 6.0 mg.

Relative Importance of Catechol-O-Methyl Transferase and Monoamine Oxidase in Metabolism of Norepinephrine

The role of MAO and catechol-O-methyl transferase in the metabolism and the inactivation of catecholamines is complex and depends on whether the catecholamine is circulating or bound, as well as on the type of species and tissues involved. Monoamine oxidase does not play a major role in terminating the activity of circulating catecholamines. It is largely responsible for intraneuronal destruction of norepinephrine and thereby regulates the levels of norepinephrine in tissues. When monoamine oxidase is inhibited, tissue catecholamine levels are increased. Drugs like reserpine or guanethidine which deplete catecholamine from its storage site, do so by releasing norepinephrine into the cytoplasm of the nerve terminal. The norepinephrine is deaminated by monoamine oxidase before it leaves the neuron. Thus, there is increased excretion of deaminnated catechols after these drugs.

Catechol-O-methyl transferase acts on norepinephrine released into the synaptic cleft as well as on circulating norepinephrine.

Uptake of Norepinephrine

Neither of these enzymes is of critical importance in the termination of the activity of norepinephrine. Inhibition of monoamine oxidase has no effect on the actions of norepinephrine, while inhibition of catechol-O-methyl transferase potentiates it. The physiological activity of catecholamines is mainly terminated by physical mechanisms, such as uptake by the axonal membrane and binding within the sympathetic neuron.

When animals are given ^{3}H-norepinephrine intravenously, plasma levels of radioactivity fall quickly. Substantial amounts of unchanged ^{3}H-norepinephrine are found in various peripheral tissues with adrenergic innervation. These results suggest that circulating catecholamines are taken up by the tissue and are retained long after physiological effects of the norepinephrine have been dissipated. Denervated tissue does not accumulate catecholamines in this way, suggesting that the site of uptake of circulating norepinephrine is the sympathetic nerve.

This uptake occurs mainly in the nerve terminals and the uptake in preterminal sympathetic fibers is very low.

The uptake and retention of catecholamines by tissue is quantitatively more important for norepinephrine than for epinephrine. Enzymatic O-methylation is more important for epinephrine.

Observations for Supporting the Uptake Theory

The uptake theory is supported by the following observations:

1. Tissue lacking a normal sympathetic innervation following surgical or chemical procedures or following immunosympathectomy loses its ability to take up and retain norepinephrine from the blood or surrounding fluid.
2. The norepinephrine taken up by the tissues innervated by sympathetic nerves can be subsequently released by nerve stimulation.
3. When sympathetically innervated tissue is depleted by

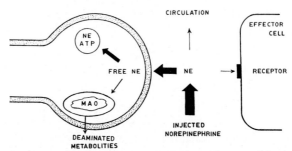

Figure 44. The effect of various drugs on the fate of injected l-norepinephrine at the adrenergic nerve terminal.

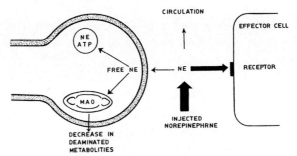

Figure 45. Schematic representation of the effect of pretreatment with cocaine on the effect of l-norepinephrine at the adrenergic nerve terminal. After administration of cocaine, transport of norepinephrine into the nerve terminal is impaired, so that more of the injected norepinephrine is available to act on the adrenergic receptors.

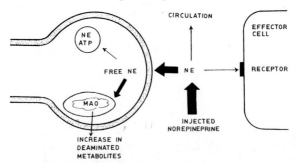

Figure 46. Schematic representation of the effect of pretreatment with reserpine or guanethidine on the fate of l-norepinephrine at the adrenergic nerve terminal. After pretreatment with reserpine or guanethidine, norepinephrine is transported into the nerve terminal at the same rate, but instead of being stored in intraneuronal vesicles, it is exposed to the action of monoamine oxidase.

reserpine, endogenous and taken-up norepinephrine disappear at the same rate.

4. Autoradiography and electron microscopy have shown that the infused norepinephrine is localized in granular vesicles.

The Relative Importance of Binding and Metabolism of Norepinephrine

In sympathetically innervated organs, catecholamines are inactivated by three mechanisms: (a) uptake and storage in nerve terminals, (b) O-methylation by catechol-O-methyl transferase, and (c) oxidative deamination by monoamine oxidase.

The estimates of the partitioning of infused norepinephrine between the various mechanisms of inactivation in perfused cat spleen, as shown in Table IX, indicates that the majority of norepinephrine is taken up by the adrenergic neuron (Fig. 44). Thus, inactivation by uptake of norepinephrine is more important than inactivation by metabolism in termination of physiological actions of circulating catecholamines. This is further supported by the fact that physiological effects of injected norepinephrine are rapidly terminated even after both the enzymes monoamine-oxidase and catechol-O-methyl transferase are inhibited.

Inactivation of Norepinephrine in Vascular Tissues

In the heart and other sympathetically innervated organs, adrenergic nerve terminals are distributed throughout the tissue, whereas in the blood vessels adrenergic nerve terminals

TABLE IX

FATE OF INFUSED NOREPINEPHRINE

Uptake by the nerves	60%
Metabolized by O-methyltransferase	15%
Interaction with receptors	5%
Overflow into the circulation (metabolized in liver)	20%

are confined to the adventitia and the adjacent portions of the media. For this reason catecholamines are inactivated differently in the vascular smooth muscles. In the adventitia and underlying media, like any other sympathetically innervated tissue, the inactivation of norepinephrine by uptake and binding seems to predominate, whereas in the greater part of the media norepinephrine is primarily inactivated not by uptake but by enzymatic breakdown.

Steps in the Uptake of Amine

Accumulation of norepinephrine into the nerve terminal involves at least two steps: (1) transport of norepinephrine across the neuronal membrane into cytoplasm of the nerve terminal, and (2) subsequent binding into the storage vesicles.

(1) *The neuron membrane uptake.* Uptake of norepinephrine across the neuronal membrane is mediated in the neuronal membrane by a carrier system which has high affinity for norepinephrine. The process is dependent on the presence of sodium ions in the external medium, the metabolic energy, and, the continual functioning of the membrane Na^+, K^+, and dependent ATPase. The carrier transports both Na^+ and amine intracellularly where carrier affinity for the amine is lowered by the low Na^+ and high K^+, thus releasing norepinephrine from the carrier into the cytoplasm of the neuron. The amine is then either stored in vesicles or deaminated by monoamine oxidase. A low physiological concentration of K^+ stimulates uptake, while high concentrations of K^+ inhibit. Neither Ca^{++} nor Mg^{++} has much influence on this uptake.

(2) *Granular uptake.* The second step in the uptake process, i.e. the intracellular concentrating mechanism, is presumably located at the granular level and requires Mg^{++}-dependent ATPase activity. This second transport mechanism is much more specific in its substrate requirement. For example, *l*-metaraminol and d-metaraminol are substrates for the neuronal membrane amine pump, but only the *l*-isomer is stored in the granules. Reserpine and low doses of guanethidine inhibit the granular uptake mechanism (Fig. 46).

Importance of Uptake

The importance of initial uptake, i.e. influx of the amine across the neuronal cell membrane, is most important for the termination of its action. Mg^{++} ATP-stimulated incorporation is physiologically important for maintaining the catecholamine content of the storage vesicles and for taking up dopamine from the cytoplasm for synthesis of norepinephrine.

The uptake of norepinephrine into nerve terminals removes the amine from the vicinity of the receptors. Normally, rapid uptake keeps the concentrations of injected norepinephrine low at the receptors. When uptake of this amine is impaired, the concentrations at the receptors on the effector organ increase, resulting in an increase in sensitivity.

When the postganglionic sympathetic fibers are transected and time is allowed for the fibers to degenerate, the tissue loses its ability to take up and retain norepinephrine (Fig. 45). This lack of uptake leads to supersensitivity. Likewise, cocaine impairs the uptake of norepinephrine and causes a similar supersensitivity. In both cases, supersensitivity is the result of availability of more amine at the receptors and not of a

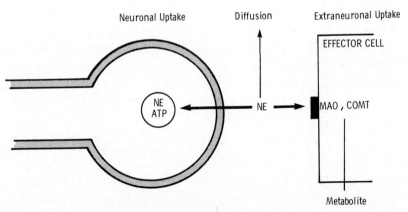

Figure 47. Schematic diagram indicating the possible site(s) of extraneuronal uptake of norepinephrine (NE).

Uptake of norepinephrine takes place into the terminal varicosities of a sympathetic neuron (neuronal uptake) and into effector cell (extraneuronal uptake).

change in the response of the effector cell to a given concentration of amine at the receptor.

Extraneuronal Uptake

In addition to the neuronal uptake of norepinephrine, another system for uptake of amine exists in various smooth muscles, cardiac muscles, and some glandular structures. The accumulation of catecholamines occurs outside of sympathetic neurons (Fig. 47), since it occurs in organs denervated either by surgical procedures or chemical methods. This extraneuronal uptake has been referred to as "uptake 2."

Extraneuronal retention of norepinephrine is a transient phenomenon. At least part of the extraneuronal norepinephrine leaves the stores without being metabolized. Therefore, it is likely that it then contributes to the concentration of amine at the receptors. The rates of extraneuronal uptake of amines are quite different from the relative rates of intraneuronal accumulation. Epinephrine, rather than norepinephrine, is a preferred amine for extraneuronal accumulation.

The pharmacological properties of extraneuronal uptake are distinct from those of neuronal uptake. For example, metaraminol or cocaine, which inhibit the neuronal uptake of norepinephrine show no effect on the extraneuronal uptake and metabolism. On the other hand, normetanephrine, methoxyamine and steroids have a greater inhibitory effect on extraneuronal accumulation and metabolism of norepinephrine. The

TABLE X
COMPARISON OF THE PROPERTIES OF NEURONAL AND
EXTRANEURONAL UPTAKE OF NOREPINEPHRINE

	Neuronal	Extraneuronal
Binding	Firm	Relatively less firm
Phenoxybenzamine	Marked inhibition	Marked inhibition
Cocaine	Marked inhibition	No effect
Normetanephrine	Slight inhibition	Marked inhibition
Metaraminal	Marked inhibition	No effect
Cold	?	Marked inhibition

comparison of extraneuronal and intraneuronal uptake is summarized in Table X.

THE PHYSIOLOGICAL FUNCTIONS OF EXTRANEURONAL UPTAKE. The physiological significance of this extraneuronal uptake is not fully known, but it is unlikely that it has any major role in the inactivation process of released and circulating norepinephrine. However, in many tissues in which the sympathetic innervation is only sparsely distributed in a large bulk of smooth muscles—for example, as in vascular smooth muscle—extraneuronal accumulation may play a role in the inactivation of released norepinephrine. This is supported by the fact that in such preparations, while inhibition of monoamine oxidase and catechol-O-methyl transferase may potentiate the response to norepinephrine and other amines, cocaine fails to do so.

Since epinephrine rather than norepinephrine is the preferred substrate for extraneuronal uptake, it is possible that this system may play some role for the rapid removal of circulating epinephrine.

CHAPTER 8

SUPRARENAL MEDULLA

THE SUPRARENAL MEDULLA is embryologically derived from the neural crest, as are the sympathetic ganglia. For this reason, the suprarenal medulla may be considered a sympathetic ganglion that has lost its axons. It follows that the innervation of the suprarenal medulla is unique because it is solely preganglionic sympathetic in nature. These preganglionic sympathetic fibers arise from the intermediolateral nucleus of T.10 through L.2 and synapse directly on the chromaffin cells which are homologues of sympathetic postganglionic neurons. After entering the sympathetic trunk, the preganglionics pass with the greater, lesser, and least thoracic splanchnic nerves and usually also with the highest lumbar splanchnics, to the celiac plexus. Without synapsing they enter the suprarenal plexus and are distributed to the chromaffin cells (Fig. 48 A&B).

There is a similarity between the cytoplasmic composition of sympathetic neurons and of suprarenal medullary chromaffin cells. The macromolecules involved in catecholamine biosynthesis and storage are similar in the two types of cells. In both types of cells catecholamines are contained in intracellular storage vesicles. Chromaffin vesicles are, however, three to five times larger than the large granular vesicles of sympathetic neurons. Vesicles from both the sympathetic neurons and the suprarenal medullary cells serve the same physiological function: to

Suprarenal Medulla

Sympathetic

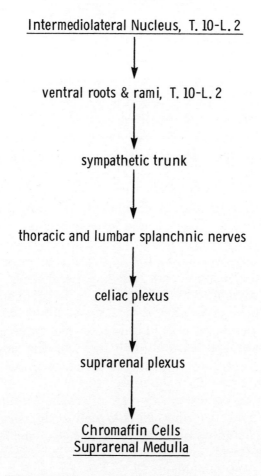

Intermediolateral Nucleus, T. 10-L. 2

↓

ventral roots & rami, T. 10-L. 2

↓

sympathetic trunk

↓

thoracic and lumbar splanchnic nerves

↓

celiac plexus

↓

suprarenal plexus

↓

Chromaffin Cells
Suprarenal Medulla

Figure 48A. Innervation of suprarenal gland.

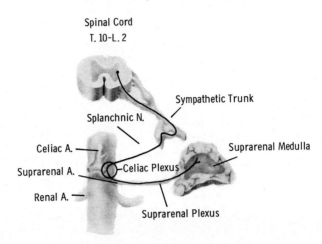

Spinal Cord
T. 10-L. 2

Sympathetic Trunk

Splanchnic N.

Celiac A.

Suprarenal Medulla

Suprarenal A.

Celiac Plexus

Renal A.

Suprarenal Plexus

SUPRARENAL GLAND

Figure 48B

synthesize, to store, and to release catecholamines in response to stimulation.

The chromaffin cells of the suprarenal medulla continuously secrete epinephrine and small amounts of norepinephrine into the blood stream. The released catecholamines reinforce the actions of all postganglionic sympathetic nerve endings except sudomotor and vasodilator. In the suprarenal medulla, norepinephrine and epinephrine are stored in specific cells. The norepinephrine-containing cells have relatively large dense-core vesicles. The relative proportion of the norepinephrine-producing and epinephrine-producing cells in this chromaffin tissue varies rather markedly with species and with age. In the adult human, roughly 80 percent of the total catecholamine content of the suprarenal medulla is epinephrine.

Under resting conditions, the rate of release of catecholamines is about 50 mμg per min per kilogram body weight. During emergency conditions such as pain, anxiety, emotional excitement, hypoglycemia and exposure to cold, the output rises from 50 to 75 mμg per minute.

Experimental studies have indicated that differential release of norepinephrine and epinephrine may be induced by different stress stimuli. For example, hypoglycemia can cause specific release of epinephrine, whereas decreased blood pressure causes the release of both amines. Rubin and Miele showed that in the cat's perfused suprarenal gland, catecholamine composition in the perfusate was a function of the duration of the stimulation. It is likely that minimal stimulation of the suprarenal medulla releases epinephrine. With more intense stimulation, epinephrine and norepinephrine are both released.

The release of epinephrine from the suprarenal medulla is important in the homeostatic control of blood glucose concentration and release of free fatty acid from adipose tissues during exercise, hypotension, asphyxia and hypoxia. The metabolic effects of catecholamines are much more pronounced with epinephrine than with norepinephrine. Epinephrine promotes the formation of cyclic 3'-5' adenosine monophosphate (Fig. 49) which stimulates glycogenolysis. Excess glucose is released from the liver and lactic acid from muscles, resulting in a rise of glucose and lactic acid (Fig. 49). Epinephrine raises the blood concentration of free fatty acid by increasing the activity of lipase, thus promoting hydrolysis of triglyceride in adipose tissue to glycerol and free fatty acid.

The suprarenal medulla is not essential for life, provided that emergency demands are minimized.

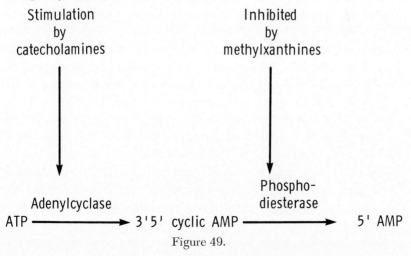

Figure 49.

CHAPTER 9

RECEPTORS

ACETYLCHOLINE AND NOREPINEPHRINE can act on a denervated organ to elicit a characteristic response. Similarly, these substances can act on the organ before it becomes innervated, for example, a four-day-old embryonic chick heart. It was this type of evidence that led to the conclusion that a released neurotransmitter does not elicit a response by acting on the nerve terminals; hence, nerves are not necessary for the organs to respond.

It is now usually believed that before a released neurotransmitter can exert its action it must unite in some way with the target cell. Specific drug-combining sites in cells have been postulated by several investigators and are referred to as receptors. The sites of various receptors are indicated in Figure 50. These postulated receptors occupy only a small portion of the cell surface. The receptors seem to be specific. Thus, acetylcholine and histamine both can cause contraction of the intestinal smooth muscle, but atropine can block the response to acetylcholine, whereas it cannot antagonize the response to histamine. This suggests that histamine is acting on a different kind of receptor. Likewise, mepyramine which antagonizes the response to histamine does not affect the response to acetylcholine.

Receptors for a particular substance are not the same in

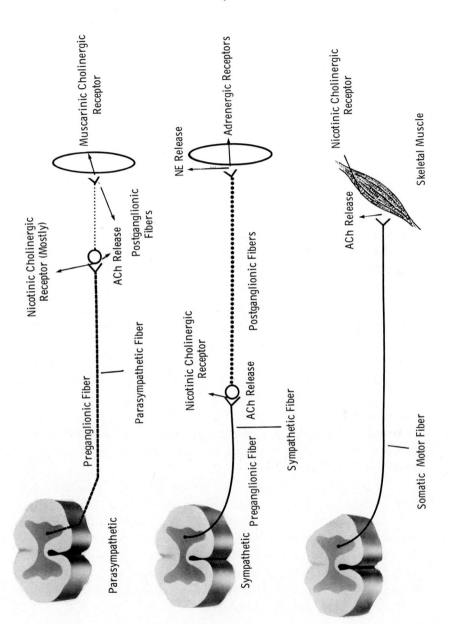

Figure 50. Sites of various receptors.

all cells. Acetylcholine action on smooth muscle, cardiac muscle and glands, but not in ganglia, can be antagonized by atropine. d-Tubocurarine, a potent inhibitor of the skeletal neuromuscular action of acetylcholine, has very little effect on its smooth muscle action and blocks ganglionic transmission only in high concentration. Furthermore, a ganglionic-blocking agent such as hexamethonium prevents the effects of acetylcholine on ganglionic transmission without blocking skeletal neuromuscular transmission. These observations suggest that receptors for acetylcholine in various tissues differ in structure and can be identified only by antagonists.

There are two main types of receptors in the autonomic nervous system. Those stimulated by acetylcholine are called cholinergic receptors, and those stimulated by norepinephrine are called adrenergic receptors.

Cholinergic Receptors

Receptors for acetylcholine are on the surface of the reactive cell because acetylcholine does not produce an effect when injected into the cell through micropipettes. Similarly, when atropine is injected into the cell, it does not antagonize the response to acetylcholine. For convenience, cholinergic receptors are subdivided into muscarinic and nicotinic receptors because muscarine and nicotine were found to stimulate them selectively. The muscarinic receptors are the atropine sensitive receptors. The nicotinic receptors are further divided into ganglionic receptors which are hexamethonium sensitive and skeletal muscle receptors which are sensitive to d-tubocurarine (Table XI). Atropine, hexamethonium, and d-tubocurarine, referred to as the antagonists, compete with acetylcholine for the binding sites in the cells. These drugs combine with the receptors without activating them. This results in a competitive blockade which can be reversed by high concentration of acetylcholine or other cholinergic drugs.

Adrenergic Receptors

In 1905, Langley proposed that there are two types of tis-

TABLE XI
RECEPTORS AT CHOLINERGIC TRANSMITTER SITES

Sites	Postganglionic	Ganglionic			Neuromuscular
Kinds of Receptors	Muscarinic	Nicotinic	*Nonnicotinic*		Nicotinic
			Muscarinic	Nonmuscarinic	
Agonists	ACh Muscarine Pilocarpine Arecoline	ACh Nicotine DMPP	ACh Pilocarpine Neostigmine McN-343 Muscarine	ACh Histamine 5-HT Angiotensin	ACh Nicotine
Antagonists	Atropine and others Belladonna alkaloids	Hexamethonium Chlorisondamine	Atropine	Cocaine Morphine	Curare

sue receptors, excitatory and inhibitory, and their response to epinephrine depends on the type of receptor with which they react. This hypothesis was supported by Dale in 1906. He found that when 0.5 mg of the active principle of ergot was injected, an intravenous administration of 200 mg of epinephrine did not cause the usual rise of blood pressure in the spinal cat. If another dose of epinephrine was given, the blood pressure did fall. Although the constrictor action of epinephrine on the blood vessels was completely antagonized by ergotoxin, the cardiac stimulatory action of epinephrine still remained. Thus, these results suggested that there are at least two sites on which epinephrine can act, one of which was blocked by administration of the active principle of ergot.

Classification of Adrenergic Receptors

It remained for Ahlquist to define clearly the concept of alpha and beta adrenergic receptors. He studied the effect of six closely related sympathomimetic amines on a variety of different systems and found differences in the order of responsiveness. In one case norepinephrine was the most active, while isoproterenol was least active. However, in other cases the order of potency was completely reversed, i.e. isoproterenol was the most active. On the basis of these findings, he postulated the existence of two types of receptors. Receptors which on stimulation cause excitatory responses are called alpha receptors. Those with an inhibitory response are called beta receptors (Table XII). In terms of circulatory response, the cardiac stimulatory activity and vasodilation produced by sympathomimetic amines were classified as beta, and vasoconstriction as alpha adrenergic responses.

Although the adrenergic receptors have not been isolated chemically, it is believed that the enzyme adenylcyclase in the cell membrane may represent at least a part of the receptor mechanism. Adenylcyclase catalyzes the formation of cyclic 3'-5' adenosine monophosphate (cyclic AMP), and it appears that cyclic AMP mediates the effects of many hormones in the body, thus acting as a second messenger.

The support for the classification of adrenergic receptors was derived from the studies with antagonists. In fact, the concept of classification of adrenergic receptors was not accepted until the discovery of dichloroisoproterenol (DCI), a derivative of isoproterenol. This drug blocked the adrenergic stimulatory effect on the heart, but did not antagonize the vasoconstriction induced by sympathomimetic amines. Since DCI antagonized those effects of adrenergic stimulation which were not blocked by ergot and which were designated by Ahlquist as beta type, DCI was classified as beta adrenergic blocking agent.

However, there are two exceptions to this classification: (a) the inhibitory effects of catecholamines on the gut which appear to be alpha responses, but are mediated by both alpha and beta receptors, and (b) the cardiac stimulatory response which is mediated entirely by beta receptors.

Drugs like phenoxybenzamine and phentolamine (α-adrenergic blocking agents) inhibit the excitatory responses of the smooth muscles and of the exocrine glands that are medi-

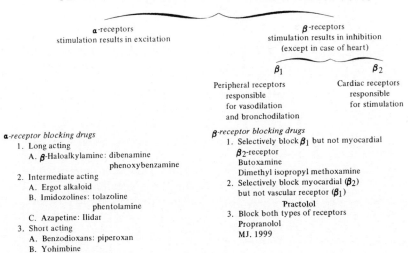

CLASSIFICATION OF ADRENERGIC RECEPTORS

α-receptors stimulation results in excitation	β-receptors stimulation results in inhibition (except in case of heart)	
	β_1	β_2
	Peripheral receptors responsible for vasodilation and bronchodilation	Cardiac receptors responsible for stimulation

α-receptor blocking drugs
1. Long acting
  A. β-Haloalkylamine: dibenamine
                 phenoxybenzamine
2. Intermediate acting
  A. Ergot alkaloid
  B. Imidazolines: tolazoline
              phentolamine
  C. Azapetine: Ilidar
3. Short acting
  A. Benzodioxans: piperoxan
  B. Yohimbine
	β-receptor blocking drugs
	1. Selectively block β_1 but not myocardial
	   β_2-receptor
	   Butoxamine
	   Dimethyl isopropyl methoxamine
	2. Selectively block myocardial (β_2)
	   but not vascular receptor (β_1)
	   Practolol
	3. Block both types of receptors
	   Propranolol
	   MJ. 1999	

TABLE XII

ated through α-adrenergic receptor stimulation. These blocking drugs, however, do not affect the following actions of
adrenergic drugs: (1) cardiac stimulation and (2) inhibitory
responses of smooth muscle.

The alpha adrenergic blockade after these drugs does not
affect the functions of sympathetic nerves or the ability of
smooth muscles to contract. Responses to circulating catechol-

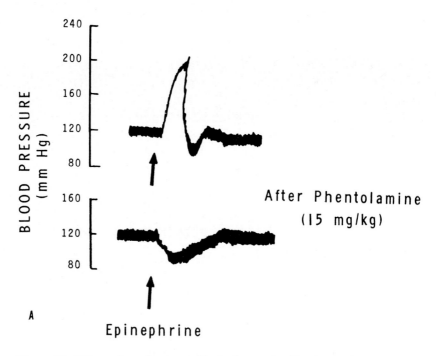

Figure 51. Effect of α-adrenergic blockade on the blood pressure response
to epinephrine. A dog was anesthetized with pentobarbital and received
1 mg/kg atropine prior to the experiment to prevent reflex bradycardia.
Injection of epinephrine caused a rise of blood pressure, which fell below
control levels before returning to normal. The epinephrine activates both
α and β receptors, but action on β-receptor is masked by the action on α
receptor. When phentolamine was injected the α-receptors were blocked.
An injection of epinephrine could then activate only β-receptor, therefore
it caused blood pressure fall. The change of the pressor response of injected epinephrine into a depressor response, is called the "epinephrine
reversal."

amines are blocked more effectively by these drugs than are responses to sympathetic nerve stimulation. This may be due to the difficulty of the drug in gaining access to the site of action of released norepinephrine. The effect produced by any of these drugs depends upon the degree of sympathetic tone which exists prior to their administration.

Alpha adrenergic blocking agents antagonize the vasopressor response to catecholamine (Fig. 51), whereas cardiostimulatory effects of catecholamines and vasodilator or bronchodilator actions of epinephrine and isoproterenol remain unaltered. These actions are mediated through stimulation of β-receptors and are antagonized by beta adrenergic blocking drugs. These beta adrenergic blocking agents exert a competitive type of blockade, i.e. there is a parallel shift of dose-response curve to the right, indicating that the antagonist (β-blocking agent) which causes the shift, is competing with the agonist (catecholamines) for a specific pharmacological receptor. Irreversible blockade as occurs with α-blocking agents has not been noticed.

Specificity of β-Blocking Drugs

Unlike α-blocking agents, β-receptor blocking drugs have a relatively high degree of specificity. For example, the cardiostimulatory response to nerve stimulation or to sympathomimetic amines is blocked by β-receptor-blocking drugs, whereas these antagonists do not block the response to other cardiostimulants, such as calcium, theophylline or digoxin. Likewise, although the vasodilation caused by isoproterenol is antagonized, the vasodilation in response to acetylcholine, nitroglycerine and histamine remains unaltered.

Classification of β-Receptors

Further development of beta-adrenoceptor agonists and antagonists have indicated that there are differences in the β-receptors of different tissues. For example, heart receptors are considered beta on the basis of selective blockade with propranolol, but norepinephrine exerts a stronger action on the beta-adrenoceptors of the heart causing an increase in both the rate and force of contraction. On the other hand, it is a very weak agonist on the beta-receptors of blood vessels in skeletal muscles. On the basis of such findings, it has been suggested that beta-adrenoceptors might be classified as at least two types. The beta$_1$-adrenoceptors include those in the peripheral system responsible for vasodilation, bronchodilation and uterine relaxation. The beta$_2$-adrenoceptors include those in the heart (and gut?). A classification of adrenergic receptors is given in Table XII. The evidence for this division is the discovery of selective beta-blocking agents. For example, N-isopropyl-methoxamine and butoxamine antagonize peripheral vasodilation in response to isoproterenol without affecting the cardiac response. On the other hand, a more recently developed drug, practolol, a cardioselective β-blocker, blocks only the β-receptors of the heart without affecting those of vascular smooth muscles and bronchi. (In certain books, the classification of β-receptors is reversed.)

The classification of the response of various effector organs to adrenergic stimuli is presented in Table XIII.

Effect of Blockade of Adrenergic Receptors on Catecholamine-Induced Glycogenolysis and Lipolysis

Catecholamines such as epinephrine cause glycogenolysis and lipolysis both *in vivo* and *in vitro*. Classification of the metabolic receptors responsible for these effects into alpha- and beta-receptors is not clear. The main difficulty is that (a) norepinephrine and epinephrine have both alpha and beta properties and (b) there are species differences in some of the metabolic responses.

GLYCOGENOLYSIS. Epinephrine stimulates adenylcyclase, an enzyme which catalyzes the formation of cyclic 3'-5' adenosine monophosphate (Fig. 52). An increase in synthesis of cyclic AMP is responsible for the glycogenolytic effect of the catecholamines. Cyclic AMP activates phosphorylase.

It has been shown that beta blockade reduces slightly the peak elevation of blood sugar caused by epinephrine and prevents a rise in lactate. On the other hand, alpha blockade reduces the rise in blood sugar by almost the same amount as does propranolol, but does not affect the rise in blood lactate. When both alpha- and beta-adrenergic receptors are blocked, the increase in blood sugar and lactate induced by epinephrine are blocked.

It seems that there are two mechanisms involved in the sympathetic control of glycogenolysis, alpha in the liver and beta in skeletal muscle.

Fat Metabolism

Catecholamines stimulate the release of free fatty acids from

TABLE XIII
CLASSIFICATION OF THE RESPONSE OF VARIOUS EFFECTOR ORGANS TO ADRENERGIC STIMULATION

Effector organ	*Receptor*	*Response*
A. *Cardiovascular System*		
Heart:		
S-A node	β_2	Tachycardia
Atria	β_2	Increased automaticity
A-V node and conducting system	β_2	Increase in conduction rate and shortening of refractory period.
Ventricle	β_2	Increased automaticity.
Blood vessels:		
Skin and mucosa	α	Constriction
Skeletal muscle	β_1	Dilation
Coronary	α and β_1	Constriction and dilation
B. *G.I. Tract*		
Motility and tone	α and β_1	Decrease
Sphincters	α	Contraction
C. *Bronchial Muscle*	β_1	Relaxation
D. *Urinary Bladder*		
Detrusor	β_1	Relaxation
Sphincter	α	Contraction
E. *Eye*		
Radial muscle, iris	α	Contraction (mydriasis)
Ciliary muscle	β_1	Relaxation
F. *Skin*		
Pilomotor muscles	α	Contraction

α-receptor and β_2 receptor stimulation results in excitatory responses, whereas stimulation of α and β_1 receptors results in inhibitory responses. The receptors in coronary arteries are controversial. It is believed that the coronary arteries have both β_1 and α-receptors. In certain books classification of β-receptors into β_1 and β_2 is reversed. It is immaterial whether one classifies β-adrenergic receptors in the heart as β_1 or β_2. The important point is that β-adrenergic receptors in the heart are different from the β-receptors in other organs.

adipose tissue, resulting in an increase in blood levels of the
fatty acid. This occurs as a result of activation of a specific
lipase in adipose tissue which then accelerates the breakdown
of triglycerides to free fatty acid.

It has been shown that catecholamine-induced lipolysis is
mediated by cyclic 3'-5' AMP. Norepinephrine and epinephrine
accelerate the rate of synthesis of cyclic AMP through stimulation of adenylcyclase (Fig. 53).

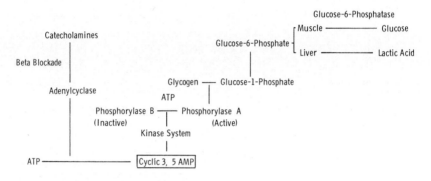

Figure 52. Schematic representation of metabolic pathways by which catecholamine stimulates glycogenolysis.

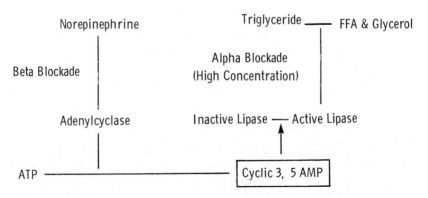

Figure 53. Schematic representation of the site of inhibition of the lipolytic
response to catecholamine by alpha and beta adrenergic blocking agents.

Both alpha and beta adrenergic blocking agents inhibit the lipolysis, though beta blockers are more potent in this regard. Recently Hynie and colleagues have shown that beta blocking agents antagonize norepinephrine-induced lipolysis mainly by interfering with the action of the amine on adenylcyclase, while alpha-blocking agents in high concentration act by direct inhibition of tissue lipase.

CHAPTER 10

SYMPATHECTOMY

W ITHIN THE LAST DECADE it has become possible to induce
sympathectomies in animals. This can be accomplished
either by injecting newborn animals with an extract containing
antibodies to nerve-growth factors (immunosympathectomy) or
by injecting animals with drugs such as 6-hydroxydopamine
(chemical sympathectomy).

Immunosympathectomy

It has long been known that certain tumors, e.g. mouse sarcoma and snake venoms, contain a factor which greatly en-
hances the growth and differentiation of sympathetic ganglia
in chick embryos. In 1954, Cohn found that the submaxillary
gland of the adult male mouse contained this factor in a concentration 6000 times greater than that in the mouse sarcoma.
This factor is a protein and is termed nerve growth factor or
NGF.

When NGF is injected daily into newborn mice, it produces
a marked increase in the volume of the sympathetic ganglia.
The effect is highly specific in the sense that no other types
of cells and, in particular, no other nerve cells are affected. The
effects of NGF on the sympathetic ganglion cells are: (a) to
increase mitotic activity, (b) to increase the number of nerve
cells, and (c) to increase the size of the nerve cells.

132

NGF is a protein and when it is injected intravenously into rabbits, antibodies to the protein are formed. If the serum from a treated rabbit is then injected into newborn mice or rats, it causes extensive destruction of the sympathetic system. This is due to the neutralization of the NGF which is essential to the development of sympathetic ganglia in newborn animals.

In sympathectomized animals, the amount of catecholamines in various organs such as the heart, spleen, etc., is very greatly reduced. There is also impairment in their capacity to take up and store norepinephrine. Sympathectomized animals can lead normal lives so long as they are not exposed to conditions of physiological stress. Sympathectomized animals have normal growth and bodily functions, such as gastrointestinal and re-reproductive. They are sensitive to cold and may have a lowered basal metabolic rate. They cannot adjust their body temperature properly when exposed to heat or low temperature. When they exhibit anger or fear, they do not show the bodily changes such as increased blood pressure or blood sugar.

Chemical Sympathectomy

6-Hydroxydopamine causes chemical denervation of adrenergic nerves. This type of denervation is similar to surgical preganglionic denervation.

Effects of Denervation on Effector Organ Responses

When preganglionic or postganglionic fibers are sectioned, the effector organs that they innervate develop a supersensitivity to transmitters and other chemical agents. The sensitivity that develops after denervation, i.e. section of the postganglionic fibers, is qualitatively different from the type of supersensitivity that develops after decentralization, i.e. section of preganglionic fibers. The mechanisms underlying the development of supersensitivity are not fully understood.

Supersensitivity after Decentralization

When preganglionic fibers are cut there is a gradual development of supersensitivity to the transmitters. This supersensitivity is probably due to some type of postsynaptic change. In the case of adrenergically innervated tissues, Trandelenburg and his colleagues have shown that supersensitivity after decentralization:

1. Is slow in onset and moderate in degree;
2. Is nonspecific so that it is as prominent with acetylcholine as it is with norepinephrine; there is a slow and gradual development of supersensitivity to all agents that stimulate normal smooth muscle;
3. May be due to an increase in receptor population or an improvement in the link between activation of receptors and contraction of the smooth muscle;
4. Is similar to that which develops after procedures which cause a prolonged interruption of the normal impulse discharge from the central nervous system to the effector organ.

Supersensitivity after Denervation

When an organ is denervated by sectioning its postganglionic fibers, certain changes occur in the effector organ. First, the nerve begins to degenerate, second, the endogenous transmitter is lost, and third, supersensitivity to the transmitter develops. The degenerating nerve terminals begin to release their transmitter. The time between the denervation and the onset of release of neurotransmitter is dependent on several factors, including the rate of axon transport in that particular nerve and the length of the axon. The release of transmitter starts generally at a time when other functions of the nerve ending are normal. The release of the transmitter is discontinuous and causes contraction of the entire smooth muscle. The effector organ then becomes subsensitive to the transmitter. This subsensitivity is transient and postjunctional. It may be due to prolonged exposure of the effector organ to the transmitter released during degeneration of the nerve terminals.

These changes occur in adrenergically as well as in cholinergically innervated organs.

In the adrenergically innervated organs, during the second day after denervation, the degenerating nerve terminals fail to take up norepinephrine and there is a rapid and pronounced increase in sensitivity to norepinephrine. This supersensitivity is most likely due to presynaptic changes, i.e. the impairment of uptake. There is no presynaptic-type supersensitivity after denervation of cholinergically innervated organs.

Since any procedure which interrupts the normal impulse traffic from the central nervous system to the effector organ causes a decentralization-type supersensitivity which is due to postsynaptic changes, and since the denervated organs likewise fail to receive tonic impulses, after forty-eight hours of denervation there is a further increase in the sensitivity of the effector organ. Thus, in adrenergically innervated organs, the denervation supersensitivity is the sum of two components: a presynaptic component due to impairment in the uptake of norepinephrine and a decentralization postsynaptic component.

CHAPTER 11

FUNCTIONAL PATHWAYS

VISUAL SYSTEM

THE AUTONOMIC NERVOUS SYSTEM is responsible for regulating the number of light rays that strike the retina and the focusing of these rays on the retina. The amount of light is controlled by constriction of pupillary muscles which regulate the diameter of the pupil. Focusing of light rays is controlled by ciliary muscles which regulate the thickness of the lens.

Innervation

The ciliary muscles are innervated solely by parasympathetic fibers. The pupillary muscles receive fibers from both autonomic divisions: the sphincter pupillae muscle from the parasympathetic and the dilator pupillae muscle from the sympathetic.

(a) Parasympathetic (Fig. 54)

The Edinger-Westphal nucleus of the oculomotor nuclear complex is the origin of the parasympathetic impulses to the eye. The preganglionic fibers are contained in the oculomotor nerve. Within the orbit these fibers travel in the inferior division of the III N. and enter the nerve to the inferior oblique muscle from which they reach the ciliary ganglion in its motor root.

Most of the preganglionic parasympathetic fibers of the III N.

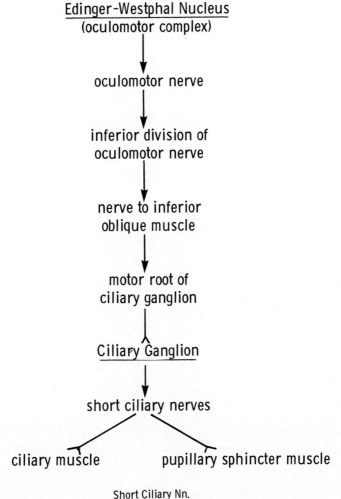

Edinger-Westphal Nucleus
(oculomotor complex)

↓

oculomotor nerve

↓

inferior division of oculomotor nerve

↓

nerve to inferior oblique muscle

↓

motor root of ciliary ganglion

↓

Ciliary Ganglion

↓

short ciliary nerves

ciliary muscle   pupillary sphincter muscle

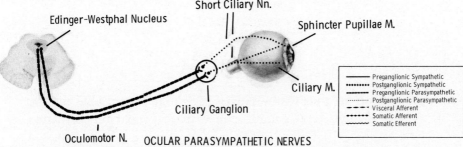

Short Ciliary Nn.

Edinger-Westphal Nucleus

Sphincter Pupillae M.

Ciliary M.

Ciliary Ganglion

Oculomotor N.   OCULAR PARASYMPATHETIC NERVES

—— Preganglionic Sympathetic
•••••• Postganglionic Sympathetic
—— Preganglionic Parasympathetic
•••••• Postganglionic Parasympathetic
– – – Visceral Afferent
•••••• Somatic Afferent
〜〜〜 Somatic Efferent

Figure 54 A and B. Parasympathetic innervation of eye.

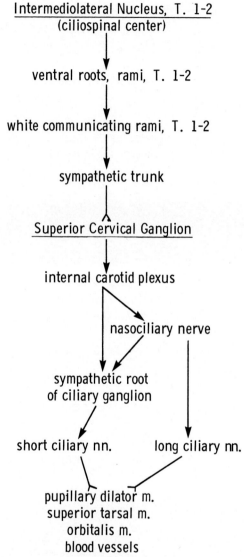

Figure 55A. Sympathetic innervation of eye.

synapse on neurons in the ciliary ganglion. (A variable number synapse in episcleral ganglia. Since these consist of postganglionic neurons that have migrated beyond the ciliary ganglion, their numbers are variable.)

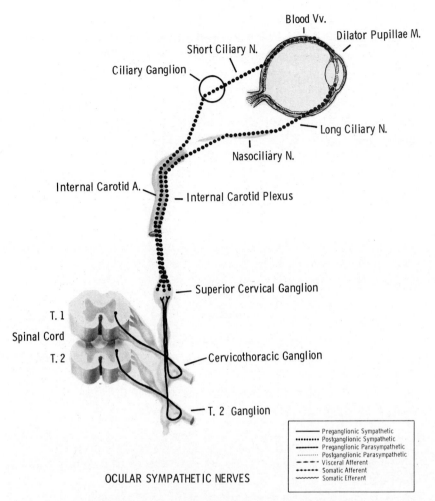

Figure 55 B. Sympathetic innervation of eye.

Postganglionic fibers from the ciliary ganglion reach the posterior part of the eyeball in the short ciliary nerves. After piercing the sclera near the optic nerve they pass anteriorly in grooves on the inner surface of the sclera. Upon reaching the ciliary body they enter and pass to the ciliary muscles and to the sphincter of the pupil.

(b) Sympathetic (Fig. 55)

Ocular sympathetic impulses originate in the ciliospinal center which consists of preganglionic neurons in the intermediolateral nucleus at spinal cord segments T. 1 and 2. The preganglionic fibers ascend in the sympathetic trunk and synapse solely in the superior cervical ganglion. Postganglionic sympathetic fibers emerge from the ganglion and travel in the internal carotid plexus and its branches to the ophthalmic plexus. Within the orbit, most of the fibers emerge from the ophthalmic plexus to join the nasociliary nerve, which then gives several long ciliary nerves to the posterior wall of the eyeball. Some postganglionic sympathetic fibers from the ophthalmic plexus travel through the ciliary ganglion *without synapsing* and reach the eye with the short ciliary nerves. The intraocular course of the postganglionic sympathetic fibers to the dilator pupillae muscle of the iris parallels the parasympathetics to the iris.

Reflexes

The autonomic regulation of the diameter of the pupil is a protective reflex phenomenon that is initiated by the intensity of light striking the eye. Regulation of the diameter of the lens is a reflex phenomenon initiated by attempts to focus on objects at different distances from the eyes.

Light Reflex (Table XIV)

The light reflex consists of constriction of the pupil upon illuminating the eye. Constriction of the ipsilateral pupil is referred to as the direct response; that of the contralateral pupil is the consensual response.

The afferent limb follows the visual pathway from the retina to the optic tract. From the optic tract these afferent impulses enter the brain stem through the brachium of the superior colliculus and synapse in the light reflex center located in the pretectal area. The pretectal neurons then send impulses bilaterally to the Edinger-Westphal nuclei, the necessary decussations occurring through the posterior commissure.

The efferent limb involves the oculomotor nerve and its

LIGHT REFLEX

Rods and Cones

Bipolar Cells

Ganglion Cells

Optic Nerve

Optic Chiasm

Optic Tract

Brachium of
Superior Colliculus

Pretectal Nuclei

Posterior Commissure

Edinger-Westphal Nuclei
of Oculomotor Complexes

Oculomotor Nerve

Inferior Division of
Oculomotor Nerve

Nerve to Inferior
Oblique Muscle

Motor Root of Ciliary Ganglion

Ciliary Ganglion

Short Ciliary Nerves

Pupillary Sphincter Muscle

TABLE XIV

branches which carry the preganglionic parasympathetic fibers to the ciliary ganglion. After a synapse here postganglionics reach the eyeball in the short ciliary nerves and travel to the sphincter pupillae muscle.

An optic nerve lesion interrupts the afferent limb and abolishes both the direct and consensual responses from the ipsila-

ACCOMMODATION AND ASSOCIATED PATHS

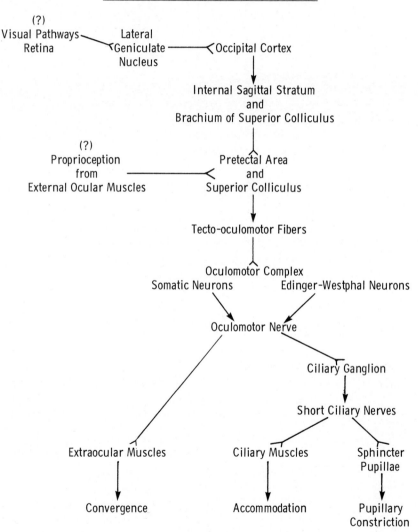

TABLE XV

teral eye. However, both pupils will react when the good eye is illuminated. An oculomotor nerve lesion interrupts the efferent limb resulting in pupillary dilatation and a loss of both the direct and consensual responses in the affected eye.

Accommodation Reflexes (*Table XV*)

When vision is changed from a distant object to a near one the light rays become more divergent upon passing through the lens. To accommodate so that the image is focused on the retina, the curvature of the lens increases. The mechanism for this accommodation is based on an inherently elastic lens that is suspended from the ciliary body. Upon contraction of its muscles, the ciliary body moves closer to the lens, thereby decreasing the tension on the suspensory ligaments. This allows the lens to increase its curvature by bulging.

To facilitate visual acuity further, convergence of the eyes and constriction of the pupils are combined with the accommodation of the lens. The reflex pathways responsible for these three phenomena are not entirely clear.

It is believed by many, that the stimulus for accommodation is the sight of an object and the reflexes are dependent upon the occipital cortex. In this case the afferent limbs in the reflexes are represented by the visual pathways from the retina to the striate cortex. Corticofugal projections from the occipital lobe then descend in the internal sagittal stratum to the superior colliculus and pretectal area.

From the accommodation center in the pretectal area and superior colliculus, impulses pass to appropriate nuclei of the oculomotor complex: the autonomic Edinger-Westphal nucleus for changes in the lens and pupil, and the somatic nuclei for convergence. The efferent limb is the oculomotor nerve with a synapse for the parasympathetic impulses (responsible for the involuntary accommodation and constriction) in the ciliary ganglion. The somatic impulses for the convergence are uninterrupted.

It has been suggested that the stimulus for accommodation is the convergence of the eyes. In this case the afferent limb of the reflex involves proprioceptive nerves in the extraocular muscles. Input from these would then influence the accommodation center in the pretectal area and superior colliculus.

There occurs in certain pathological conditions, such as tabes dorsalis resulting from syphilis or tumors near the posterior part of the third ventricle, an Argyll Robertson sign which is characterized by a small pupil that does not react to light but does react well on accommodation. The underlying mechanism is not understood and has not been localized. The loci most frequently considered are centrally, in the rostral part of the pretectal area or peripherally, in the iris itself.

Physiology of the Iris and Ciliary Muscles

Iris

Constriction of the pupil (miosis) is elicited by contraction of the sphincter pupillae muscle of the iris. The iris is a contractile circular diaphragm that forms the colored part of the eye and controls the amount of light reaching the retina. When excessive light enters the eye, the circular muscles are reflexly stimulated resulting in constriction of the pupil, thereby reducing to a reasonable degree the amount of light that strikes the retina.

Dilatation of the pupil (mydriasis) is elicited by a decrease in constrictor muscle tone or an increase in dilator muscle tone. The latter is regulated by sympathetic nerves and occurs with contraction of the dilator pupillae muscle of the iris. When the radial muscles are stimulated, there is dilatation of the pupil without a loss of accommodation and constriction of the intraocular blood vessels and vessels of the conjunctiva.

Ciliary Muscle

The lens is attached to the ciliary muscle by a series of strands called the ciliary zonule or the suspensory ligament of the lens. When the eye is at rest, the lens is kept in a flattened state because of the tension exerted by the ligament and the eye is accommodated for far vision. The ciliary body contains smooth muscles innervated by parasympathetic nerves from the ciliary ganglion. Contraction of this muscle moves the ciliary body forward, thereby releasing the tension on the suspensory ligament and the lens assumes its natural spherical shape. The eye is then accommodated for near vision. Thus, accommodation for near vision is dependent on the ability of the ciliary muscles to contract. When the parasympathetic system is impaired, there is a loss of accommodation (cycloplegia), i.e., distant vision remains good, but near vision is indistinct.

Associated Phenomena

Intraocular Pressure

The aqueous humor is contained in the anterior and posterior chambers of the eye. It is secreted into the posterior chamber from the epithelium covering the ciliary body. It passes through the pupil into the anterior chamber and drains through the filtration angle into the canal of Schlemm. When the pupil is dilated, it narrows the ciliary angle restricting the drainage of the aqueous humor. Since secretion continues, intraocular pressure rises. Drugs which produce dilatation of the pupil may produce an increase in intraocular pressure, especially in patients predisposed to glaucoma. The drugs which cause pupillary constriction, when instilled in the eye, diminish the intraocular pressure by drawing the smooth muscle of the iris away from the canal of Schlemm, thereby establishing better drainage of the aqueous humor.

Horner's Syndrome

Interruption of sympathetic impulses to the orbit produces pupillary constriction, ptosis, dilatation of the orbital vessels, and enophthalmos. These phenomena are associated with Horner's syndrome and occur through lesions either centrally, located in the brain stem or cervical spinal cord, or peripherally, located in the sympathetic system.

Effects of Drugs

Cholinergic Drugs

Acetylcholine-like drugs such as pilocarpine, carbachol or an anticholinesterase such as eserine, produces miosis and accommodation for near vision. Drugs which block the muscarinic actions of acetylcholine such as atropine and hyoscine and those which block parasympathetic ganglia, e.g. hexamethonium and mecamylamine, cause dilatation of the pupil and paralyze accommodation. Intraocular pressure is aggravated. Therefore they are contraindicated in glaucoma.

Adrenergic Drugs

Sympathomimetic drugs such as ephedrine or phenylephrine produce dilation of the pupil by increasing the sympathetic activity. They do not paralyze the accommodation, though they may limit the range.

Clinical Use

1. Drugs which produce dilatation of the pupil (mydriasis) are used to aid in the examination of the retina. In diagnostic work atropine is used, but homoatropine is preferred since mydriasis and cycloplegia produced by a single application of atropine can last up to ten days.

Some physicians prefer sympathomimetic drugs to dilate the pupil since there is no loss of accommodation and since actions of amine are of short duration.

2. Atropine-like drugs are useful in treatment of inflammatory states such as acute iritis and keratitis (inflammation of the cornea), since prolonged mydriasis is useful because of the enforced relaxation of the iris.

3. In treatment of inflammation of the conjunctiva due to congestion of the blood vessels, sympathomimetic drugs are useful.

HEART

Although the heart is abundantly supplied by parasympathetic, sympathetic, and afferent nerves it can function in the absence of all extrinsic nerves as is seen in the case of the transplanted heart.

Parasympathetic

Cardiac parasympathetic preganglionic fibers arise from the dorsal nucleus of the vagus nerve and synapse on postganglionic neurons scattered in the cardiac plexus and epicardium, and along the conducting system. Branches from the cervical parts of the vagus nerves carry preganglionic parasympathetic fibers to the cardiac plexus through the cervical sympathetic cardiac nerves, whereas branches from the thoracic parts of the vagus nerves pass directly to the cardiac plexus. The cardiac ganglia consist of postganglionic parasympathetic neurons located extrinsically in the cardiac plexus, or intrinsically in the epicardium and along the conducting system. Postganglionic fibers from these ganglion cells synapse in the sinu-atrial (SA) and atrioventricular (AV) nodes. The right vagus nerve innervates the SA node and right atrium and produces slowing of the heart. The left vagus nerve innervates the AV conduction tissue and can cause heart block. There is no parasympathetic nerve supply to the ventricles (Fig. 56).

Sympathetic

Cardiac sympathetic preganglionic fibers arise from the intermediolateral nucleus of T.1 to 4 (perhaps T.5 & 6 also) and synapse on postganglionic neurons in all of the cervical and the upper four to six thoracic trunk ganglia. Postganglionic fibers travel through the superior, middle, and inferior cervical cardiac nerves and also the thoracic cardiac nerves to join the cardiac plexus. They are distributed to the sinu-atrial and atrioventricular nodes, the coronary arteries, and the myocardium.

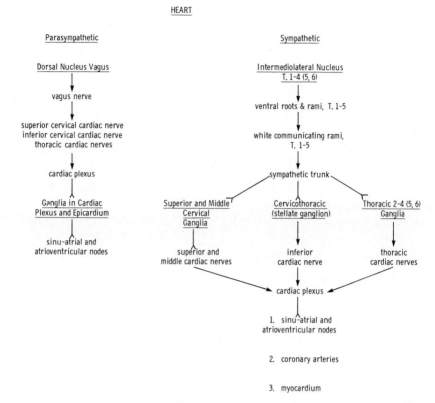

Figure 56A. Innervation of heart.

Afferent Nerves

Visceral afferent impulses arising from the heart course in the vagus and sympathetic nerves. Those from receptors that are stimulated by increased pressure, ascend in the vagus nerves. The neuronal cell bodies are located in the inferior (nodose) ganglion and they synapse centrally in the nucleus solitarius. Reflex connections with medullary vasomotor and cardio-inhibitory centers result in a lowering of the blood pressure and a decrease in heart rate.

Impulses from receptors in the adventitia of the coronary arteries and the connective tissue of the heart travel mainly in the left cervical and thoracic cardiac nerves to the sympathetic trunk. These visceral afferent fibers reach the upper

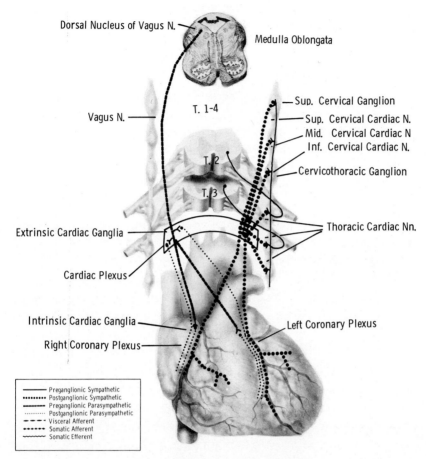

Figure 56B. Innervation of heart.

thoracic spinal nerves through the appropriate white communicating rami. Their cell bodies are in the upper four or five thoracic dorsal root ganglia and they synapse centrally in the upper thoracic segments of the spinal cord. These connections are the anatomical basis for the cardiac pain referred to the left side of the chest and the inner aspect of the left arm.

Physiology

The heart has its own inherent rhythm. The frequency and

strength of the heart beat is regulated by the autonomic nerves. The neurohumoral control is illustrated in Figure 57.

Stimulation of the vagi cardiac nerves causes release of acetylcholine (Auch) which produces the following:

1. Decreased heart rate;
2. Decreased atrial contractility and hence ventricle filling; it does not affect ventricular contractility. Therefore, there is a consistent decrease in cardiac output;
3. Decreased coronary blood flow;
4. Prolongation of AV conduction time; therefore, the effective refractory period of the conduction system is increased;
5. Complete ventricular rest (intense stimulation). If stimulation continues, the ventricle once again begins to contract, i.e. vagal escape occurs;
6. A continuous discharge of impulses passes via the vagus to the heart to maintain tone. Thus, tone in the heart is vagal. The degree of vagal tone varies with muscular training; therefore, athletes have slow pulses. When vagal impulses are interrupted, heart rate increases to twice that of the initial rate.

Stimulation of the sympathetic cardiac nerves causes:

1. Increased rate and force of contraction;
2. Increased oxygen consumption and coronary blood flow;
3. Shortened effective refractory period and conduction time of the atrial muscle, atrioventricular node and ventricular muscle;
4. Atrial contractions toward the end of the right ventricle diastole. The increase in the force of atrial contractions causes an increase in the pressure within the ventricle and thereby increases the degree of stretching of the myocardium before contraction. Starling's curve states that in the individual muscle fiber, the tension developed on contraction is a function of the initial length before contraction. Applying this relationship to myocardial fibers, a more effective contraction should therefore result from

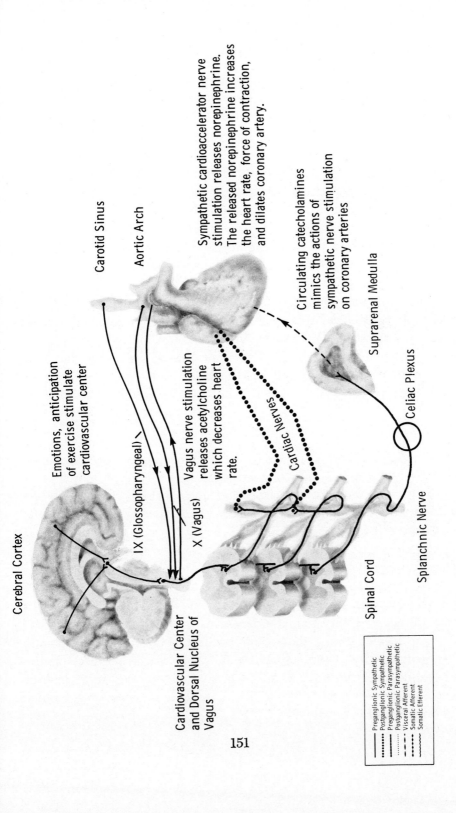

Cerebral Cortex

Carotid Sinus

Aortic Arch

Sympathetic cardioaccelerator nerve stimulation releases norepinephrine. The released norepinephrine increases the heart rate, force of contraction, and dilates coronary artery.

Circulating catecholamines mimics the actions of sympathetic nerve stimulation on coronary arteries

Suprarenal Medulla

Celiac Plexus

Emotions, anticipation of exercise stimulate cardiovascular center

IX (Glossopharyngeal)

X (Vagus)

Vagus nerve stimulation releases acetylcholine which decreases heart rate.

Cardiac Nerves

Spinal Cord

Splanchnic Nerve

Cardiovascular Center and Dorsal Nucleus of Vagus

Preganglionic Sympathetic
Postganglionic Sympathetic
Preganglionic Parasympathetic
Postganglionic Parasympathetic
Visceral Afferent
Somatic Afferent
Somatic Efferent

a greater degree of stretching of fibers by increased filling pressure: ↑ *atrial contraction* → ↑ *ventricle filling* → ↑ *pressure within ventricle* → ↑ *diastolic fiber length* → improved systolic *tension*. Stimulation of the sympathetic cardiac nerves also shifts the length tension curve to the left, i.e. greater contractility for the same initial length.

Thus, sympathetic stimulation increases the contractility in these four ways:

1. By increasing the atrial contractility and hence initiating stretch of the ventricle muscle fiber;
2. By acting directly on the ventricle and moving its length tension curve to the left;
3. By increasing the coronary blood flow;
4. By increasing cardiac output which may increase the blood pressure. The rise in blood pressure may in turn reflexly increase the vagal tone and reverse or mask the local sympathetic effects on the heart.

ALIMENTARY CANAL

The first and last parts of the alimentary canal are controlled by voluntary nerves and reflexes, e.g. voluntary muscles for suckling, muscles of mastication and deglutition, and the external anal sphincter. The parts from the esophagus to the anus receive innervation from both the parasympathetic and sympathetic systems. The preganglionic neurons of the parasympathetic system are in the dorsal nucleus of the vagus and in the sacral intermediolateral nucleus whereas the postganglionic neurons are in the myenteric and submucous plexuses. In the case of the sympathetic nerves, the preganglionic neurons are located in the thoracolumbar intermediolateral cell column, whereas the postganglionic neurons are in the plexuses on the abdominal aorta (celiac, superior mesenteric, and inferior mesenteric) and internal iliac arteries (superior and inferior hypogastric plexuses).

Esophagus (Table XVI)

Parasympathetic

Preganglionic vagal fibers arise from the dorsal nucleus of the vagus nerve, enter the esophageal plexus from the cervical branches of the vagus and synapse on ganglion cells in the myenteric and submucous plexuses. Postganglionic parasympathetic fibers from the myenteric and submucous ganglia supply the muscular coats and glands of the esophagus.

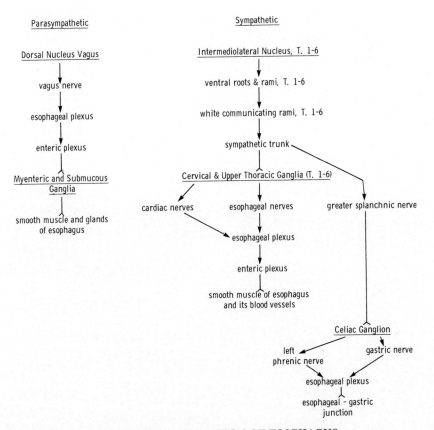

TABLE XVI. INNERVATION OF ESOPHAGUS.

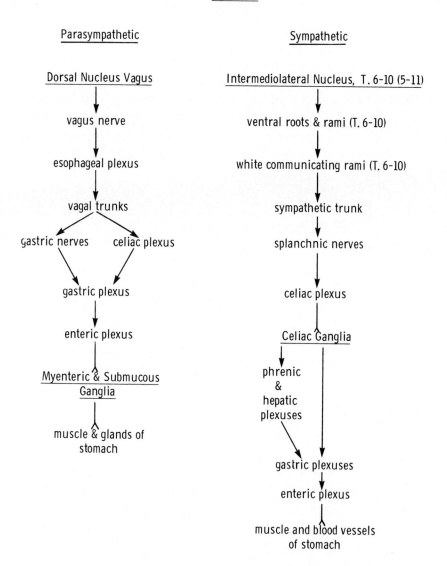

Figure 58A. Innervation of stomach.

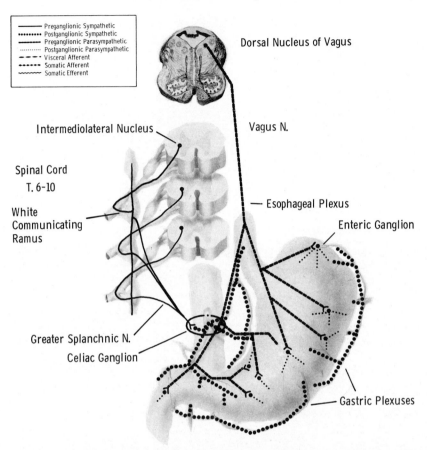

Figure 58b. Innervation of stomach.

Sympathetic

Preganglionic sympathetic fibers arise from the intermediolateral nucleus of T.1 to 6 and synapse mostly in the cervical and upper thoracic trunk ganglia; some preganglionics synapse in the celiac ganglion. Postganglionic fibers from the cervical and upper thoracic trunk ganglia travel in their cardiac and esophageal branches to the esophageal plexus on the surface of the esophagus. After entering the esophagus they supply the blood vessels and smooth muscle either directly or after cours-

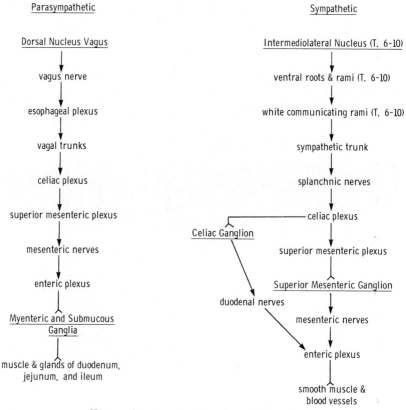

Figure 59a. Innervation of small intestine.

ing through the enteric plexuses. Those postganglionic sympathetic fibers that originate in the celiac ganglion innervate the lowest part of the esophagus (esophageal–gastric junction) from the left phrenic and gastric nerves.

Stomach (Fig. 58)

Parasympathetic

The gastric preganglionic parasympathetic fibers descend in the vagus nerves to the esophageal plexus and enter the abdomen in the vagal trunks. Without synapsing, these pre-

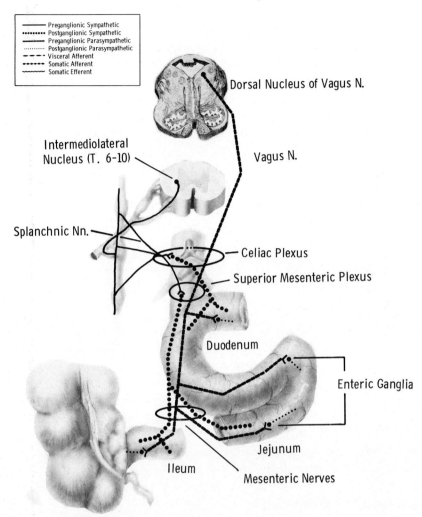

Preganglionic Sympathetic
Postganglionic Sympathetic
Preganglionic Parasympathetic
Postganglionic Parasympathetic
Visceral Afferent
Somatic Afferent
Somatic Efferent

Dorsal Nucleus of Vagus N.

Intermediolateral
Nucleus (T. 6-10)

Vagus N.

Splanchnic Nn.

Celiac Plexus

Superior Mesenteric Plexus

Duodenum

Enteric Ganglia

Jejunum

Ileum

Mesenteric Nerves

Figure 59. Innervation of small intestine.

ganglionic fibers reach the gastric plexus through the celiac plexus and gastric nerves. After entering the wall of the stomach, they join the enteric plexuses and synapse on neurons in the myenteric and submucous ganglia. Postganglionic parasympathetic fibers from these ganglia innervate the gastric musculature and glands.

Sympathetic

The gastric preganglionic sympathetic fibers arise from the intermediolateral nucleus from about T.6 to T.10 and synapse in the celiac ganglion. After entering the sympathetic trunk from the white communicating rami of spinal nerves T.6 to 10, they emerge mainly in the greater splanchnic nerves and pass to the celiac plexus. After synapsing in the celiac plexus, they enter the gastric plexuses either directly or after traversing the phrenic and hepatic plexuses. Within the wall of the stomach they supply the gastric musculature and blood vessels either directly from the perivascular plexuses or after entering the enteric plexuses.

Small Intestine (Fig. 59)

Parasympathetic

The preganglionic parasympathetic fibers that influence the duodenum, jejunum, and ileum pass from the dorsal nucleus of the vagus to the intestinal enteric ganglia. After descending in the esophageal plexus and entering the abdomen in the vagal trunks, these preganglionics traverse the celiac and superior mesenteric plexuses (without synapsing). They reach the wall of the small intestine by following the mesenteric plexuses that are located along the mesenteric arteries. Within the small intestine these preganglionic parasympathetic fibers synapse on neurons in the myenteric and submucous plexuses. Postganglionic fibers from these enteric ganglia innervate the muscular coats and intestinal glands.

Sympathetic

The duodenal, jejunal, and ileal preganglionic sympathetic fibers come from the intermediolateral nucleus of T.6 to 10 and synapse in the celiac and superior mesenteric ganglia. These preganglionics traverse the sympathetic trunks (without synapsing) and travel in the greater splanchnic nerves to the celiac and superior mesenteric plexuses. After synapsing in the celiac ganglion, duodenal postganglionic sympathetic fibers travel a perivascular route along the duodenal branches of the celiac artery. Those postganglionic sympathetic fibers destined for the jejunum and ileum synapse in the superior mesenteric ganglion and travel along the perivascular mesenteric nerves. Within the wall of the small intestine the postganglionic sympathetics innervate the blood vessels and intestinal muscles either directly or after entering the enteric plexuses.

The components of the enteric plexuses are illustrated in Figure 60.

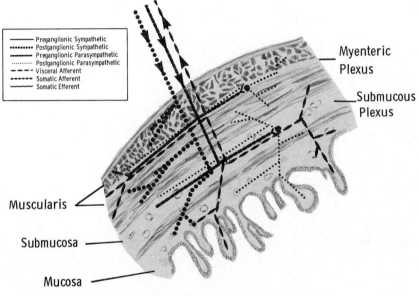

Figure 60. Components of enteric plexuses.

Large Intestine and Rectum (Fig. 61)

Parasympathetic

The large intestine has a dual parasympathetic nerve supply, i.e. from both cranial and sacral parts. The enteric ganglia of the cecum and the ascending and transverse parts of the colon receive preganglionic parasympathetic fibers from the dorsal nucleus of the vagus nerve. These preganglionic vagal

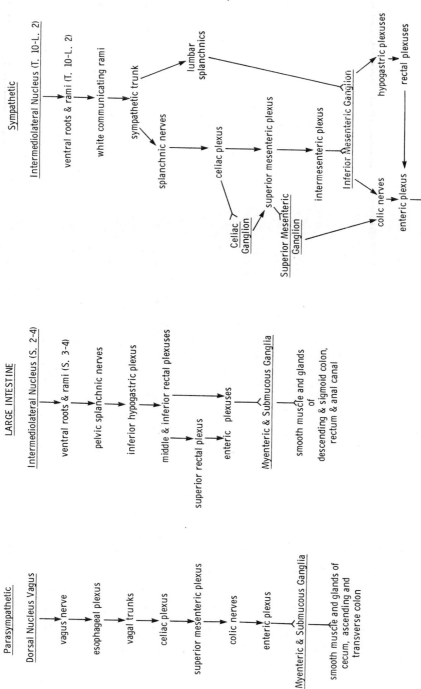

Figure 61a. Innervation of colon and rectum.

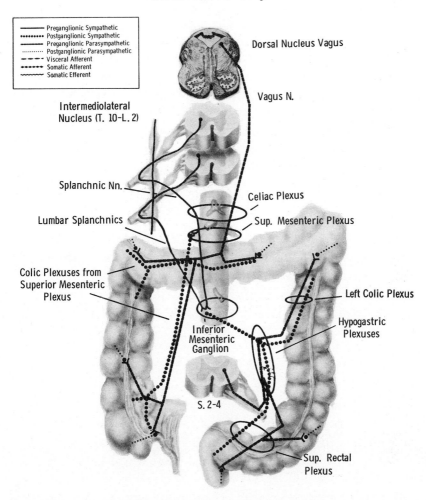

Preganglionic Sympathetic
Postganglionic Sympathetic
Preganglionic Parasympathetic
Postganglionic Parasympathetic
Visceral Afferent
Somatic Afferent
Somatic Efferent

Dorsal Nucleus Vagus

Vagus N.

Intermediolateral
Nucleus (T. 10–L. 2)

Splanchnic Nn.

Celiac Plexus

Lumbar Splanchnics

Sup. Mesenteric Plexus

Colic Plexuses from
Superior Mesenteric
Plexus

Left Colic Plexus

Inferior
Mesenteric
Ganglion

Hypogastric
Plexuses

S. 2-4

Sup. Rectal
Plexus

Figure 61b. Innervation of colon and rectum.

fibers descend in the esophageal plexus, enter the abdomen in
the vagal trunks, and then course (without synapsing) to the
celiac and superior mesenteric plexuses. They reach the cecum
and the ascending and transverse colons by passing along the
colic branches of the superior mesenteric plexus. The descending and sigmoid parts of the colon as well as the rectum receive
preganglionic parasympathetic fibers from the intermediolateral
nucleus of S.2 to 4. These preganglionics enter the pelvic

cavity in the pelvic splanchnic nerves, join the inferior hypogastric plexus, and reach the descending and sigmoid parts of the colon through the left colic plexus or more commonly as independent retroperitoneal nerves. These parasympathetic components come from the hypogastric plexuses and join other components (sympathetic and afferent) coming from the inferior mesenteric plexus.

Preganglionic parasympathetic fibers reach the rectum mainly in the middle rectal plexus which arises from the upper part of the inferior hypogastric plexus. Fibers from the middle rectal plexus ascend to join the distal parts of the superior rectal plexus.

Upon entering the walls of the large intestine and rectum, the preganglionic parasympathetic fibers enter the enteric plexuses and synapse in the myenteric and submucous ganglia. Postganglionic parasympathetic fibers from these intrinsic ganglia innervate the smooth muscles and glands of the large intestine and rectum.

Sympathetic

Preganglionic sympathetic fibers for the large intestine and rectum arise from the intermediolateral nucleus of T.10 through L.2 and synapse in the celiac and the superior and inferior mesenteric ganglia. Some preganglionics reach the inferior mesenteric ganglion directly from the lumbar splanchnic nerves. Other preganglionics come from the thoracic splanchnics and descend through the celiac, superior mesenteric, and intermesenteric plexuses. Postganglionic sympathetics from the celiac and superior mesenteric ganglia reach the cecum and the ascending and transverse parts of the colon through the colic nerves which travel along the colic branches of the superior mesenteric artery. Postganglionic sympathetics from the inferior mesenteric ganglion reach the descending and sigmoid parts of the colon through the left colic plexuses (branches of the inferior mesenteric), the upper part of the rectum through the superior rectal plexus (also from the inferior mesenteric), and the lower part of the rectum through the middle rectal plexus (which arises from the inferior hypogastric plexus).

Physiology of Alimentary Canal

The gastrointestinal tract has its own intrinsic neural control, but both the parasympathetic and sympathetic nerves affect its activity, the parasympathetic especially.

Physiologically effective anabolic activity of the gastrointestinal tract requires the glandular release of digestive secretions and rhythmic contractions. The parasympathetic system provides the stimulus required for these digestive processes. Thus, stimulation of the parasympathetic nerves causes: (1) an increase in the contractility, motility, and tone of the stomach and intestines; (2) a relaxation of the junctional sphincters (cardiac, pyloric, and ileocecal sphincters) to allow movement of food and residue along the enteric pathway; and (3) enhancement of glandular secretions. Not all the glands of the gastrointestinal tract are stimulated. (The glands are not entirely controlled by nerves.)

Sympathetic stimulation has an opposite effect: there is a decrease in the contractility, motility and tone of the digestive tract, contraction of the sphincters, and inhibition of gastric secretion during sympathetic stimulation. During emergency situations the sympathetic nervous system becomes active and inhibits the anabolic or vegetative activities of the digestive tract. Thus, all the digestive activities are postponed until the emergency is over.

BRONCHI AND LUNGS

The smooth muscle of the respiratory tree is innervated by both sympathetic and parasympathetic fibers (Fig. 62).

Parasympathetic

Preganglionic parasympathetic fibers arising from the dorsal nucleus of the vagus nerve, reach the pulmonary plexuses through the bronchial branches of the vagus, and synapse on

BRONCHI AND LUNGS

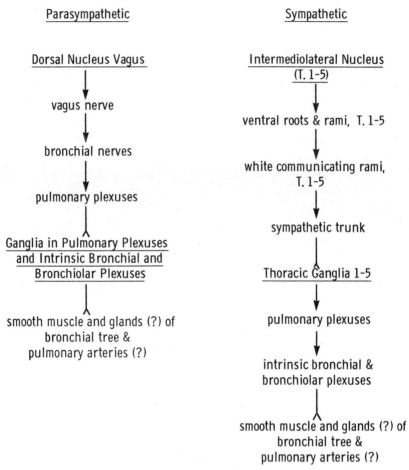

Figure 62a. Innervation of bronchi and lungs.

ganglia in the pulmonary, bronchial, and bronchiolar plexuses. Postganglionic fibers accompany the bronchial and bronchiolar plexuses and innervate the smooth muscle of the respiratory tree and blood vessels.

Sympathetic

Preganglionic sympathetic fibers from the intermediolateral nucleus of T.1 to 5 synapse in the sympathetic trunk ganglia

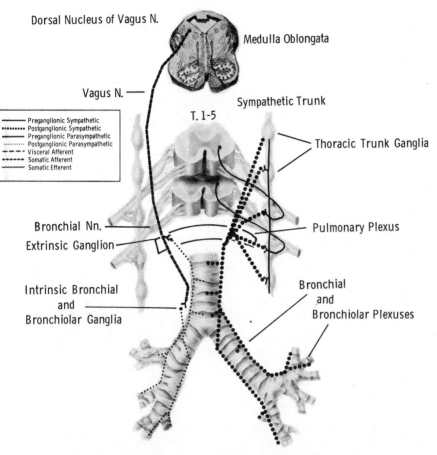

Figure 62b. Innervation of bronchi and lungs.

at the same levels. Postganglionic fibers from these upper five thoracic ganglia enter the posterior pulmonary plexus and are distributed via the intrinsic bronchial and bronchiolar plexuses to the smooth muscle of the respiratory tree and pulmonary blood vessels.

Afferent Nerves

Visceral afferent impulses from receptors in the visceral pleura, in the adventitia of the pulmonary vessels, and mainly in the walls of the bronchioles and bronchi travel in the vagus nerves. All cell bodies are in the inferior (nodose) ganglia and they synapse centrally in the nucleus solitarius. Reflex connections are made with medullary respiratory and vasomotor centers. Those endings stimulated by stretching of the lungs during inspiration are concerned with the reflex control of respiration. The endings in the mucous membrane of the bronchi initiate the cough reflex.

Physiology

The autonomic system plays little or no role in respiration since inhalation and exhalation of air is a function of somatic nerves and the voluntary muscles of the diaphragm and thoracic wall.

Stimulation of sympathetic nerves produces dilatation of the bronchi and bronchioles and constriction of the pulmonary blood vessels, thereby reducing mucous secretion. Parasympathetic stimulation has quite the opposite effect. It causes constriction of the bronchi and bronchioles and possibly an increase in secretion of the bronchial glands.

Usually autonomic effects on the bronchi and lungs go unnoticed. However, in persons with asthma, these effects become pronounced and adrenergic drugs, such as ephedrine, epinephrine, and isoproterenol, which mimic sympathetic stimulation, are used effectively in the treatment of the asthmatic. Likewise, drugs such as atropine which block the effects of acetylcholine on muscarinic receptors, are constituents of the preparations used in the treatment of asthma in cases where bronchodilator and antisecretory actions are helpful.

BILIARY SYSTEM, PANCREAS, AND SPLEEN

Stimulation of biliary and pancreatic parasympathetic nerves produces muscular contraction of the gall bladder and bile ducts, relaxation of the sphincters, and exocrine secretion in the pancreas. The preganglionic parasympathetic fibers arise in the dorsal nucleus of the vagus and synapse on intrinsic ganglion cells (Fig. 63 A,B,&C). The preganglionics descend in the esophageal plexus and enter the celiac plexus in the vagal trunks. Without synapsing in the celiac plexus, some preganglionics enter the hepatic plexus to reach the intrinsic ganglion cells in the walls of the gall bladder and bile ducts. Other preganglionics pass through the superior mesenteric and pancreatic plexuses to synapse on intrinsic pancreatic interlobar ganglia. Postganglionic fibers from these intrinsic ganglia innervate the smooth muscle of the gall bladder and bile ducts and the exocrine glands of the pancreas.

Stimulation of biliary, hepatic, pancreatic, and splenic sympathetic nerves causes constriction of the blood vessels of these organs. Preganglionic sympathetic fibers originate from the intermediolateral nucleus of T.6 to 10 and synapse in the celiac or superior mesenteric ganglia which they reach via the splanchnic nerves. Postganglionic sympathetics are distributed to the hepatic and splenic plexuses from the celiac ganglia and to the pancreatic plexus from the celiac and superior mesenteric ganglia.

URINARY SYSTEM

Sympathetic nerves innervate the blood vessels of all parts of the urinary system and the trigonal muscle of the urinary bladder. Parasympathetic nerves innervate only the detrusor muscle of the bladder and the smooth muscle of the ureter (Fig. 64 A,B&C).

Sympathetic

Sympathetic preganglionic fibers arise from the intermediolateral nucleus of T.10 through L.2 and synapse on postganglionic neurons in the celiac and hypogastric plexuses and in the lumbar sympathetic trunk. After entering the sympathetic trunk those preganglionics that influence the renal vasculature pass via the splanchnic nerves to ganglion cells in the celiac plexus. Postganglionic fibers from the celiac ganglion travel via the renal plexus to the blood vessels of the kidney and

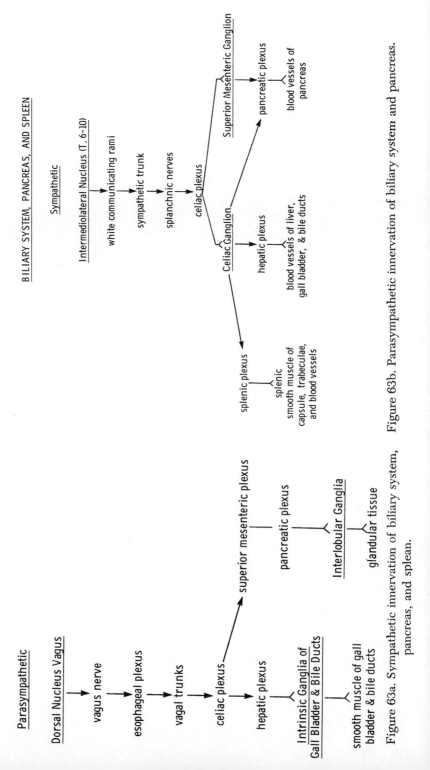

Figure 63b. Parasympathetic innervation of biliary system and pancreas.

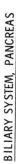

Figure 63a. Sympathetic innervation of biliary system, pancreas, and splean.

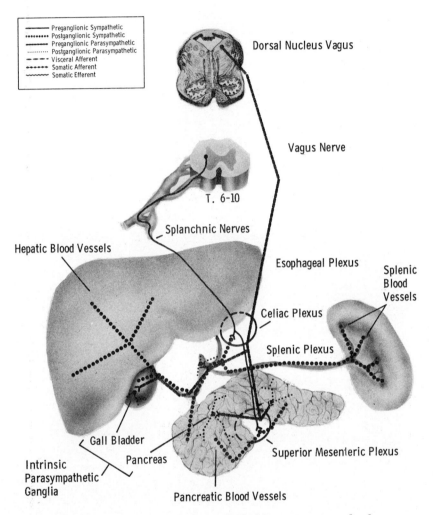

Figure 63C. Innervation of liver, gall bladder, pancreas and spleen.

upper ureter. Some preganglionic sympathetic fibers that control the trigonal muscle and blood vessels of the bladder and lower ureter emerge in the lumbar splanchnic nerves, course through the inferior mesenteric plexus, and synapse on ganglion cells in the hypogastric plexuses. Other preganglionics synapse in the lumbar trunk ganglia. Postganglionics pass through the

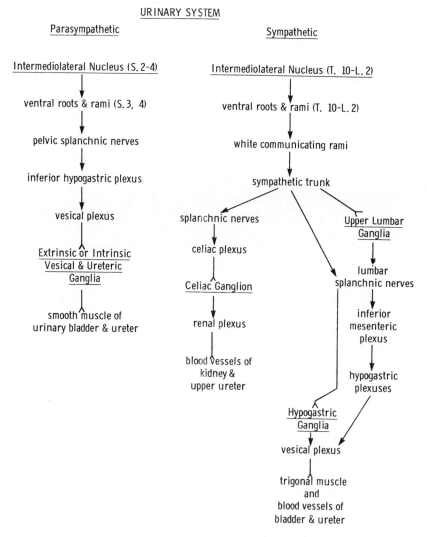

Figure 64a. Innervation of urinary system.

lumbar splanchnics, inferior mesenteric plexus, and hypogastric plexus to the vesical plexus. From the vesical plexus, post-ganglionics from the lumbar trunk and hypogastric ganglia innervate the trigonal muscle of the bladder and the blood vessels of the bladder and lower ureter.

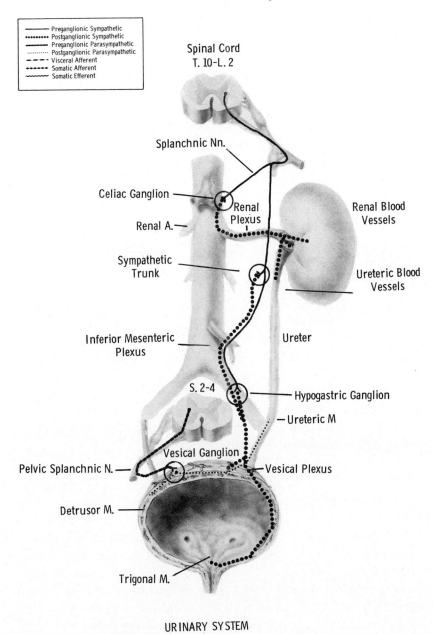

Figure 64B. Innervation of urinary system.

Parasympathetic

The parasympathetic preganglionic fibers arise from the intermediolateral nucleus of S.2 to 4, enter the pelvic cavity through the pelvic splanchnic nerves and join the inferior hypogastric plexus which carries them into the vesical plexus. They synapse on postganglionic neurons either in the vesical plexus or in the walls of the bladder and ureter. Axons from these extrinsic or intrinsic terminal ganglia are the postganglionic fibers that innervate the detrusor and the muscular walls of the ureter.

Afferent Nerves

Visceral afferent impulses arising from the urinary organs course to the spinal cord via sympathetic and parasympathetic paths. Those from the kidney and upper ureter pass exclusively via sympathetics and have their cell bodies located in the spinal ganglia of T.11 through L.1. The lower ureter and bladder send sympathetically-routed impulses via the spinal ganglia of T.11 through L.2 and parasympathetically-routed impulses via the spinal ganglia of S.2 to 4. An exception to the general rule that the pain impulses follow the sympathetic nerves occurs in the case of pain from the neck of the bladder which passes with the pelvic splanchnic nerves and enters the spinal cord through the dorsal roots of S.2 to 4.

Physiology of Urination

Excitation of parasympathetic nerves causes contraction of the detrusor muscle of the bladder which results in increased intravesicle pressure. Stimulation of sympathetic nerves causes contraction of the trigone and is thought to be related to ejaculation. The parasympathetic system is more important in controlling bladder function than the sympathetic system. After removal of parasympathetic nerves urination is impossible. The bladder becomes distended and urine always dribbles, and there is never a complete emptying of the bladder.

In addition to autonomic nerves, somatic motor nerves also

participate in the activity of the urinary system. The external sphincter, or sphincter urethrae, is comprised of striated muscle and is innervated by the perineal branch of the pudendal nerve; hence, it is under voluntary control.

Although controversy still exists, the current concept is that micturition is initiated by voluntary relaxation of the pelvic floor, including the external sphincter. The mechanism involves relaxation of that part of the pelvic diaphragm that supports the neck of the bladder so that the resistance in the urethra decreases allowing urine to flow if the vesicle pressure is high enough. Cessation of urination is brought about by voluntary contraction of the pelvic diaphragm that supports the neck of the bladder. Thus, autonomic nerves play no role in initiation or cessation of urination.

REPRODUCTIVE SYSTEM
Male

The male sex organs receive sympathetic fibers that mainly innervate the walls of the ejaculatory system and parasympathetic fibers that control the erectile tissue of the penis (Fig. 65).

Sympathetic

Sympathetic preganglionic fibers arise from the intermediolateral nucleus of T.10 through L.2 and synapse on postganglionic neurons in the intermesenteric and inferior mesenteric plexuses. After entering the sympathetic trunk the preganglionics pass, without synapsing, through the thoracic splanchnic nerves, celiac, superior mesenteric, and intermesenteric plexuses to ganglion cells scattered in the intermesenteric, inferior mesenteric, or hypogastric plexuses. Postganglionics to the blood vessels of the testis travel from the intermesenteric ganglia along the testicular plexus. Those components of the testicular plexus destined for the epididymis and wall of the proximal part of the ductus deferens arise from the inferior mesenteric or superior hypogastric ganglia. The smooth muscle of the distal

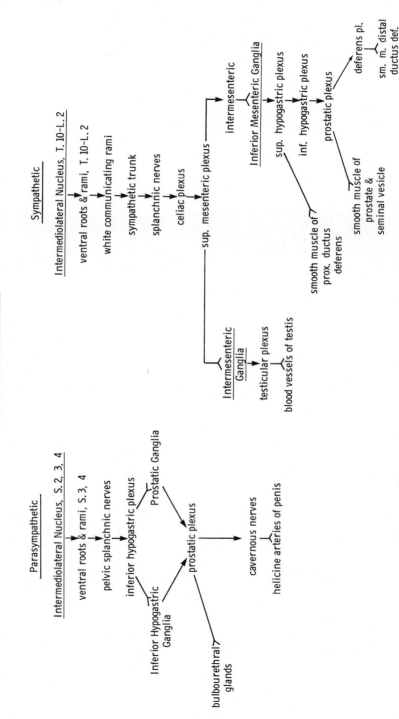

Figure 65a. Innervation of male reproductive system.

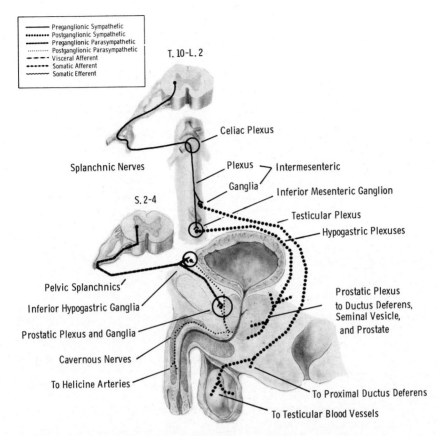

Figure 65B. Innervation of male reproductive system.

part of the ductus deferens as well as that of the prostate gland and seminal vesicle receive postganglionic fibers from inferior mesenteric and hypogastric ganglia via the vesical and prostatic plexuses.

Parasympathetic

The parasympathetic preganglionic fibers arise from the intermediolateral nucleus of S.2–4, enter the pelvic cavity in the pelvic splanchnic nerves and synapse on pelvic ganglia in the inferior hypogastric and prostatic plexuses. Postganglionic fibers then continue forward from the prostatic plexus as the cav-

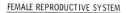

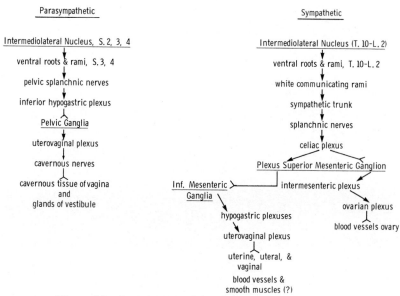

Figure 66a. Innervation of female reproductive system.

ernous nerves to the helicine arteries in the cavernous tissue of the penis.

Afferent Nerves

Visceral afferent impulses arising from the male sex organs pass to the spinal cord via sympathetic and parasympathetic paths. Those following sympathetic nerves have their cells located in the spinal ganglia of T.10 through L.2; those running with parasympathetic nerves are found in the spinal ganglia of S.2 to 4. An exception to the general rule that visceral pain impulses follow the sympathetic nerves occurs in the case of pain from the prostate, which travels in the pelvic splanchnics to enter the cord through the dorsal roots of S.2 to 4 (where the parasympathetic impulses arise).

Female

The female sex organs receive sympathetic fibers that innervate the blood vessels of all organs and the muscular walls of

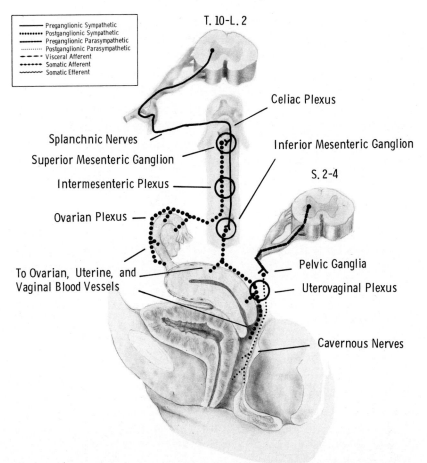

Figure 66B. Innervation of female reproductive system.

the uterus and uterine tube. The parasympathetic nerves influence the cavernous tissue of the vagina and the glands of
the vestibule (Fig. 66).

Sympathetic

The sympathetic preganglionic fibers arise from the intermediolateral nucleus of T.10 through L.2 and synapse on
postganglionic neurons located either in the superior and inferior mesenteric ganglia or in the lower lumbar and the
sacral trunk ganglia. After entering the sympathetic trunk

some preganglionics emerge in the thoracic splanchnic nerves, traverse the celiac plexus without synapsing, and enter the superior mesenteric plexus. Some preganglionics synapse here; postganglionic fibers then traverse the intermesenteric plexus to the ovarian plexus and are distributed to the ovarian blood vessels and upper part of the wall of the uterine tube. Other preganglionic fibers traverse the superior mesenteric and inter-mesenteric plexuses to synapse in the inferior mesenteric ganglion. Postganglionics from here reach the uterovaginal plexus via the hypogastric plexuses. Other sympathetic postganglionics reach the uterovaginal plexus by traveling from the lower lumbar and sacral sympathetic trunk ganglia via the pelvic splanchnic nerves. Uterine and vaginal branches of the uterovaginal plexus innervate the blood vessels and smooth muscle of the uterus and lower part of the uterine tube, and the vagina, respectively.

Parasympathetic

The parasympathetic preganglionic fibers arise from the intermediolateral nucleus of S.2–4, enter the pelvic cavity in the pelvic splanchnic nerves and synapse on pelvic ganglia in the inferior hypogastric and uterovaginal plexuses. Postganglionic fibers then course in the cavernous nerves to cavernous tissue of the vagina and the glands of the vestibule.

Afferent Nerves

Visceral afferent impulses arising from the female sex organs course to the spinal cord via the sympathetic and parasympathetic paths. Those following sympathetic nerves have their cells located in the spinal ganglia of T.10 through L.2, whereas those running with the parasympathetic nerves are found in the spinal ganglia of S.2 to 4. An exception to the general rule that visceral pain fibers follow the sympathetic nerves occurs in the case of pain from the cervix of the uterus which travels in the pelvic splanchnic nerves and enters the cord through the dorsal roots of S.2–4 (where the parasympathetic impulses arise).

Physiology of Reproductive System

The parasympathetic nerves innervate the cavernous tissues of the penis and clitoris. Erection occurs as a result of arterial dilatation and venous compression. This phenomenon allows blood to enter the cavernous tissues under a high pressure. Stimulation of the pelvic parasympathetic nerves produces dilatation of the helicine arteries thereby causing engorgement of the erectile tissue. The veins become compressed thus hindering venous return and aiding erection.

Stimulation of the pelvic parasympathetic nerves also causes secretion of accessory reproductive glands (cervical and vestibular in the female and prostate, seminal vesicle, and bulbourethral in the male) to provide the necessary lubricants for coitus.

Afferent impulses from erotogenic areas excite the preganglionic parasympathetic neurons associated with erection. Superimposed on this basic reflex arc are the influences of impulses from higher centers in the brain by means of which other types of stimuli, e.g. visual, olfactory, can cause erection. Likewise, stimuli acting through association areas of the brain can exert an inhibitory effect on the erection reflex. This inhibitory effect can prevent the occurrence of erection or abolish it once it has begun. This inhibitory mechanism is frequently the cause of impotence. Subsidence of erection may also occur from stimulation of the sympathetic nervous system. Erections presumably on a hormonal basis without involving spinal cord or higher center participation, also occur.

When the stimuli mediating erection are sufficiently intense they set up a series of nervous and muscular effects culminating in orgasm during which there is ejaculation of semen in the man and rhythmic muscular contractions of the distended vagina in the woman. The orgasm produces a general excitatory effect on the sympathetic system resulting in increased heart rate, blood pressure, and metabolic rate, as well as an increase in respiration.

Sympathetic stimulation results in the ejaculation of semen by the contractions of the smooth muscle of the ductus deferens and ejaculatory ducts accompanied by somatic nervous stimulation of appropriate voluntary muscles (bulbospongiosus). Section of the sympathetic nerves leads to the inability to ejaculate. Likewise, just as higher brain centers can cause impotency by inhibiting erection, they also can cause impotency by inhibiting ejaculation.

Except for their blood vessels, the ovary, the testis, and the uterus do not respond to stimulation of autonomic nerves.

AUTONOMIC INNERVATION OF LIMBS

The blood vessels, sweat glands, and arrector pili muscles of the limbs are innervated by postganglionic sympathetic nerves that reach the limbs either via the brachial and lumbosacral plexuses or by traveling with the major blood vessels supplying each limb (see Fig. 13).

Upper Limb (Table XVII).

Vasomotor, sudomotor, and pilomotor sympathetic fibers travel to the upper limb mainly by way of the brachial plexus. The preganglionic neurons are located in the intermediolateral cell column from approximately T.2 to T.9 or 10. After reaching the sympathetic trunks via the appropriate white communicating rami they ascend and synapse in ganglia located higher up.

Postganglionic sympathetic fibers arising mainly from the cervicothoracic ganglion and in part from the vertebral and second and third thoracic ganglia travel via the gray communicating rami to the ventral rami of C.7 and 8 and T.1. An intrathoracic ramus, the nerve of Kuntz, connects the first and second thoracic nerves (and sometimes the second and third).

A small number of postganglionic fibers from the cervicothoracic and second thoracic ganglia pass through vascular filaments to the subclavian artery and are distributed along its branches to the more proximal parts of the upper limb.

Lower Limb (Table XVIII)

Vasomotor, sudomotor, and pilomotor sympathetic fibers

UPPER LIMB

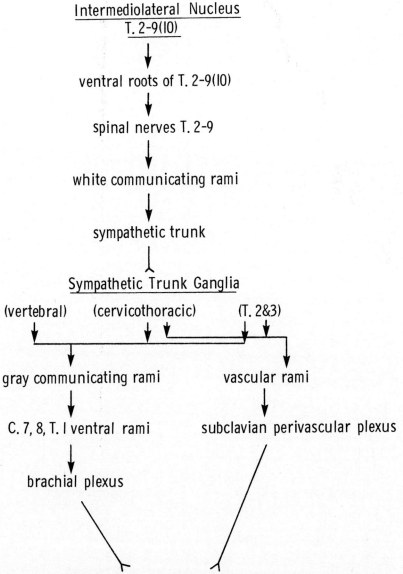

Intermediolateral Nucleus
T. 2-9(10)

↓

ventral roots of T. 2-9(10)

↓

spinal nerves T. 2-9

↓

white communicating rami

↓

sympathetic trunk

Sympathetic Trunk Ganglia

(vertebral)   (cervicothoracic)   (T. 2&3)

gray communicating rami   vascular rami

C. 7, 8, T. I ventral rami   subclavian perivascular plexus

brachial plexus

blood vessels, sweat glands, arrector pili muscles

TABLE XVII. INNERVATION OF UPPER LIMB.

LOWER LIMB

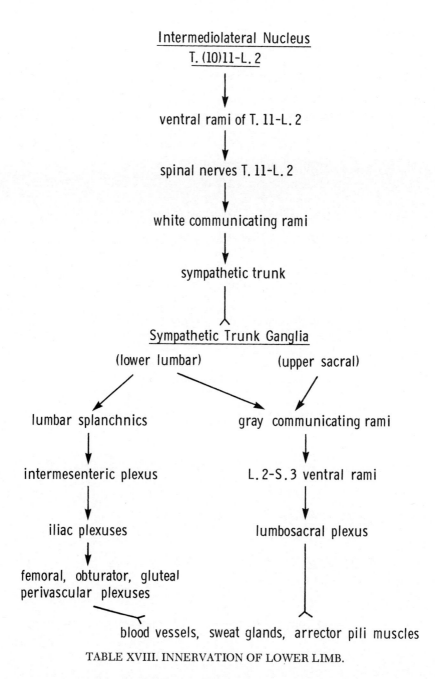

TABLE XVIII. INNERVATION OF LOWER LIMB.

travel to the lower limb mainly by way of the lumbosacral plexus. The preganglionic neurons are located in the intermediolateral cell column from approximately T.11 through L.2. After reaching the sympathetic trunk through the appropriate white communicating rami they descend to ganglia located lower down.

Postganglionic sympathetic fibers arising from the lower lumbar and upper two or three sacral ganglia travel via gray communicating rami to the ventral rami that form the roots of the lumbosacral plexus.

A small number of postganglionic fibers from the lumbar ganglia pass via the lumbar splanchnic nerves to the intermesenteric plexus surrounding the aorta. These reach the more proximal parts of the lower limb in the perivascular plexuses surrounding the branches of the iliac arteries. Other postganglionic fibers reach the femoral and obturator arteries from the respective nerves. In addition, a small number of postganglionic fibers from the upper two or three sacral ganglia pass via the tibial nerve to the popliteal artery and are distributed with its branches to the leg and foot.

CHAPTER 12

PHARMACOLOGY OF AUTONOMIC DRUGS

NEURAL TRANSMISSION is highly vulnerable to the actions of drugs (Fig. 67). Drugs exert their effects by modifying one or more stages in neurohumoral transmission. In addition, drugs may have properties which are unrelated to their action on neurotransmission.

Drugs may act (1) on the presynaptic sites to alter the storage of, synthesis of, or the release of neurotransmitters; and (2) on the postsynaptic site(s) to mimic, potentiate, or antagonize the actions of neurotransmitters. It is possible for a drug to have multiple sites of action (Fig. 68).

Drugs Acting on Cholinergic Synapses

A. *Drugs Acting on Presynaptic Sites* (Fig. 69)
  1. *Drugs altering the rate of synthesis*
     Drugs like hemicholinium affect the rate of synthesis by interfering with a choline transport mechanism. Triethylcholine inhibits the synthesis by interfering with acetylation of acetylcholine. Triethylcholine may be incorporated instead of choline. The acetic ester of triethylcholine is stored instead of acetylcholine and may impair synaptic transmission.

184

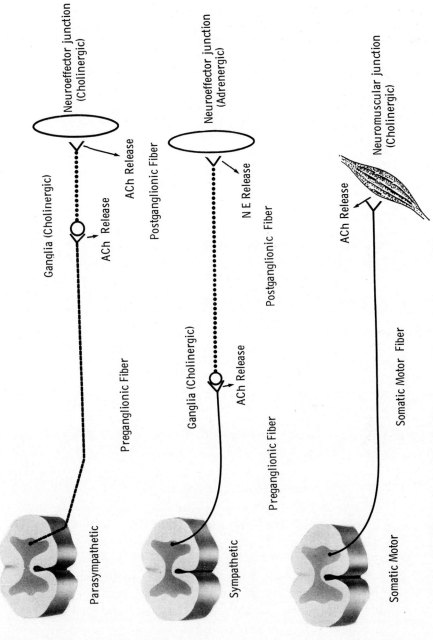

Figure 67. Locations and sites of action of cholinergic and adrenergic drugs.

Drugs exert their effects by modifying one or more of the steps or stages of neurohumoral transmission. In addition, a drug may have properties which are unrelated to its action on neurotransmission.

Site of Action

Drugs can act at:

1. ganglia
2. neuroeffector junction
3. neuromuscular junction

Mode of Action

Drugs may act at:

1. presynaptic sites to alter the rate of synthesis or release of neurotransmitter
2. postsynaptic sites to mimic, potentiate, or antagonize the actions of neurotransmitter
3. both sites

Pharmacologic Classification of Drugs

There are two categories:

1. adrenergic drugs
2. cholinergic drugs

Figure 68.

2. *Drugs altering the rate of release*
   Toxins like botulinum and ions like Mg^{++} inhibit the release of acetylcholine, whereas Ca^{++} ions enhance this release.
B. *Drugs Acting at Postsynaptic Sites* (Fig. 70)
   Acetylcholine is the transmitter (a) at motor end-plates, (b) at postganglionic parasympathetic nerve terminals, and (c) at both parasympathetic and sympathetic preganglionic nerve terminals in ganglia.

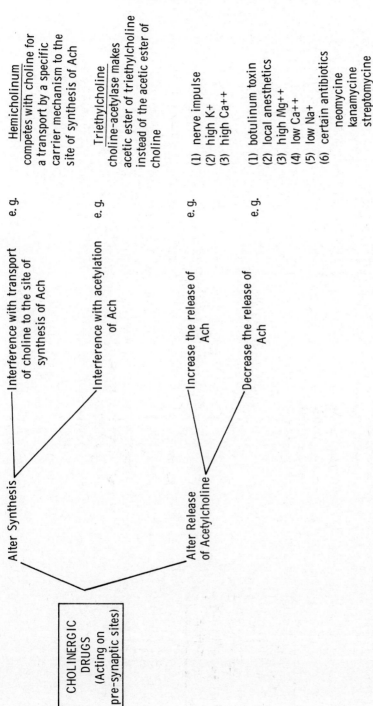

CHOLINERGIC DRUGS (Acting on pre-synaptic sites)

Alter Synthesis

Interference with transport of choline to the site of synthesis of Ach

e. g. Hemicholinum competes with choline for a transport by a specific carrier mechanism to the site of synthesis of Ach

Interference with acetylation of Ach

e. g. Triethylcholine choline–acetylase makes acetic ester of triethylcholine instead of the acetic ester of choline

Alter Release of Acetylcholine

Increase the release of Ach

e. g. (1) nerve impulse
(2) high K+
(3) high Ca++

Decrease the release of Ach

e. g. (1) botulinum toxin
(2) local anesthetics
(3) high Mg++
(4) low Ca++
(5) low Na+
(6) certain antibiotics
    neomycine
    kanamycine
    streptomycine

These drugs act by altering the rate of synthesis or release of acetylcholine (Ach) at pre-synaptic sites. They are not of therapeutic importance.

Figure 69.

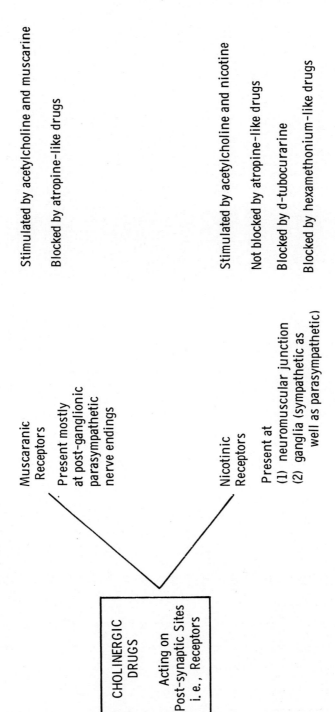

Figure 70.

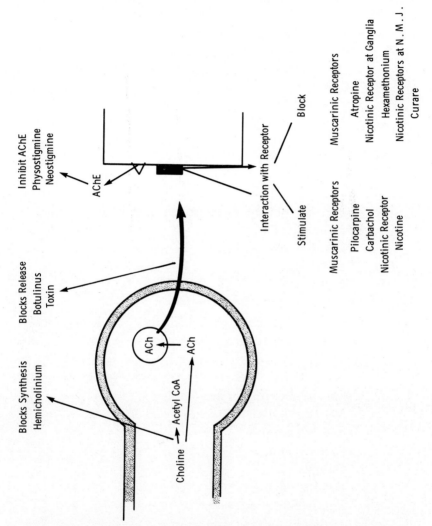

Figure 71. The sites of action of some drugs modifying transmission at cholinergic synapse.

1. *Drugs mimicking the action of transmitters*
A drug occupying the specific cholinergic receptors may activate them and is called a depolarizer. Such drugs, therefore, share affinity as well as intrinsic activity. Since the receptors at cholinergic synapses differ there are different drugs for each type of receptor. Examples are:
   a. *Neuromuscular junction*
      Choline esters
      Nicotine
      Phenyltrimethylammonium (PTMA)
   b. *Ganglia*
      Nicotine
      Dimethylphenylpiperazinium (DMPP)
   c. *Neuroeffector sites*
      Choline esters (such as carbachol)
      Pilocarpine
      Muscarine
2. *Drugs blocking the receptors*
Drugs may interact with receptors preventing acetylcholine or related drugs from activating them, i.e., they share the affinity with acetylcholine but lack its intrinsic activity. Such drugs are antagonistic to acetylcholine and examples are:
   a. *Neuromuscular junctions*
      d-Tubocurarine
      Succinylcholine
   b. *Ganglia*
      Hexamethonium
   c. *Neuroeffector sites*
      Atropine and related drugs
3. *Drugs potentiating the effect of released acetylcholine*
Drugs like physostigmine or neostigmine potentiate the effect of released acetylcholine. They cause inhibition of the enzyme cholinesterase which is responsible for hydrolysis of acetylcholine thereby allowing acetylcholine to accumulate.

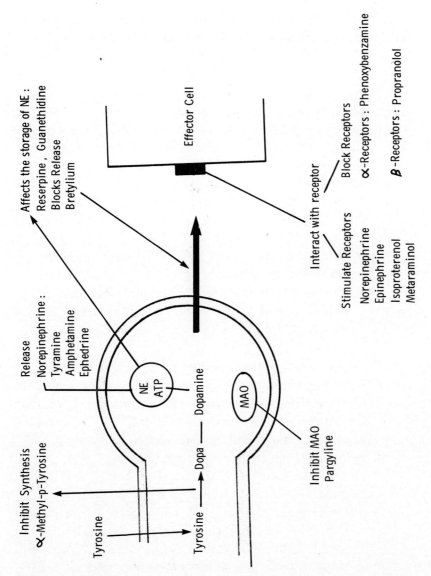

Figure 72. The sites of action of some drugs modifying transmission at adrenergic synapse.

The site of action of some drugs modifying transmission at the cholinergic synapse is presented in Figure 71.

Drugs Acting on Catecholamine Synapses

A. *Drugs Acting on Presynaptic Sites*
  1. *Drugs altering the rate of synthesis*
     Compounds like alpha-methyl-para-tyrosine may inhibit the conversion of tyrosine to dopa by competing with the tyrosine.
  2. *Drugs replacing the neurotransmitter*
     a. Some sympathomimetic amines such as tyramine and amphetamine may act indirectly by displacing the norepinephrine stores mole by mole. This released norepinephrine reacts with receptors causing sympathomimetic effects.
     b. Drugs such as metaraminol or alpha-methyl norepinephrine may replace the norepinephrine in the storage granules so that less norepinephrine is released (See Fig. 24).
  3. *Drugs affecting the granular storage mechanism*
     Reserpine or guanethidine may deplete norepinephrine by interfering with granular storage mechanism so that the norepinephrine cannot be stored and is therefore exposed to the action of monoamine oxidase.
  4. *Drugs affecting the neuronal membrane*
     Drugs may interfere with transport into or out of the neuron:
     a. Drugs may interfere with the uptake of the norepinephrine, which consequently would result in more norepinephrine at the receptors. Such drugs will cause potentiation to exogenous and released norepinephrine, e.g. cocaine, imipramine, and guanethidine.
     b. Drugs may block the transport of norepinephrine out of the membrane, e.g. chlorpromazine.
  5. *Drugs affecting the adrenergic fiber*
     Drugs such as bretylium interfere with the physiologic

release of norepinephrine from the adrenergic fiber without depleting its catecholamine.

6. *Drugs interfering with enzymatic destruction*

The monoamine oxidase inhibitors, e.g. pargyline, protect the intraneuronally released norepinephrine from inactivation and, therefore, cause an increase in intraneuronal catecholamine content. The increased catecholamine content can inhibit the norepinephrine synthesis by a feedback mechanism.

B. *Drugs Acting On Postsynaptic Site(s)*

1. *Drugs mimicking the actions of neurotransmitters*

Drugs may activate the receptors and may cause responses similar to norepinephrine, but not as efficiently as norepinephrine, e.g. octopamine, metaraminol.

2. *Drugs blocking the receptors*

Drugs may interact with the receptors, preventing norepinephrine from activating them, and thereby depressing the response to the released physiologic transmitter, e.g. phenoxybenzamine, propranolol.

The site of action of some drugs modifying transmission at the adrenergic synapse is shown in Figure 72.

INDEX

195